PRAISE FOR LOST CHILDREN

Rachelle offers insight and reassurance for those who have suffered miscarriage, and guidance for those desiring to comfort their loved ones. She emphasizes that we are all children of a loving Heavenly Father, despite the trials we face.

—Richard Paul Evans

In a religion centered on the family unit, challenges with fertility and pregnancies are often cause for even more heartbreak and uncertainty. The title of this book, for me, had a double meaning: lost children in reference to the prayed-for children we are unable to raise due to miscarriage or inability to conceive, but also in reference to parents who might feel they have become lost children to their Father in Heaven. It is so difficult to have faith in a plan that sometimes leaves us wounded to our core. Rachelle Christensen has done a wonderful job of not only honestly telling her story, but gathering generations' worth of information that helps lead us to our own understanding of the trials we as women often face in our goal of having a family. Beautifully written and tactfully approached, *Lost Children* is a wonderful resource for those women whose hearts are broken and provides assistance for those aching to offer comfort in a situation that often seems comfortless.

Any woman who has lost a child and felt that she too has been lost along the way, will find comfort, security, and hope within the pages of this book.

—Josi S. Kilpack,
author of *Unsung Lullaby*

As a licensed professional counselor, I've had the privilege of working with many people over the past twenty-eight years, and I've always found the most challenging situations are those involving good people trying to cope with the personal loss of a loved one. I believe the saddest cases are those involving a miscarriage. In her book, *Lost Children: Coping with Miscarriage for Latter-day Saints*, author Rachelle Christensen offers help to those who have suffered with this tragedy, as well as rendering sound advice for those wanting to help, but who are not sure what to do or say.

Written through the experience of having endured the heartbreak of a miscarriage, Ms. Christensen guides the reader through an empathic trail of understanding and hope. Filled with the reassurance offered by the gospel of Jesus Christ, Ms. Christensen helps us understand God's greater picture and the security and love which is found in trusting Him to make all things right in the end.

Lost Children: Coping with Miscarriage is one of those high quality reference books that belongs on every therapist's bookshelf. It is an excellent gift for every woman who has been called upon to endure such a deep, personal loss. Additionally, Church leaders will find this book to be a great source of understanding into the needs and pains of women struggling with a miscarriage.

I intend to utilize this book in my practice and highly recommend it as a source of help and comfort. Anyone who reads her compassionate account will gain insights into this area of emotional and personal tragedy which is all too often neglected.

—Russell Beck, LPC &
Licensed Designated Examiner
for the State of Utah

As a woman who has gone through miscarriage herself, author Rachelle Christensen knows what she's talking about. With facts, gospel insight, experience, and compassion, *Lost Children* provides understanding and help to those coping with the very real emotions that accompany miscarriage. It is a wonderful resource not only for those who have had a miscarriage, but also for those who have a loved one dealing with it.

—Jaime Theler, author of
Enjoying the Journey and coauthor of
Parenting the Ephraim's Child

LOST
c·h·i·l·d·r·e·n

COPING WITH MISCARRIAGE
for LATTER-DAY SAINTS

Also by Rachelle J. Christensen

Wrong Number

.

LOST
c·h·i·l·d·r·e·n

COPING WITH MISCARRIAGE
for LATTER-DAY SAINTS

R. J. Christensen

With a Foreword by W. Lawrence Warner, MD

CFI
Springville, Utah

This is not an official publication of The Church of Jesus Christ of Latter-day Saints. The opinions and views expressed herein belong solely to the author and do not necessarily represent the opinions or views of Cedar Fort, Inc. Permission for the use of sources, graphics, and photos is also solely the responsibility of the author.

ISBN 13: 978-1-59955-248-4

Published by CFI, an imprint of Cedar Fort, Inc., 2373 W. 700 S., Springville, UT 84663
Distributed by Cedar Fort, Inc. www.cedarfort.com

LIBRARY OF CONGRESS CATALOGING-IN-PUBLICATION DATA

Christensen, Rachelle J., 1978-
  Lost children : coping with miscarriage / Rachelle J. Christensen.
     p. cm.
  Includes bibliographical references.
  ISBN 978-1-59955-248-4 (acid-free paper)
  1. Miscarriage--Religious aspects--Church of Jesus Christ of Latter-day
Saints. 2. Stillbirth--Religious aspects--Church of Jesus Christ of
Latter-day Saints. 3. Bereavement--Religious aspects--Church of Jesus
Christ of Latter-day Saints. I. Title.

  BX8643.D4C57 2009
  248.8'66--dc22

       2009006456

Cover design by Angela D. Olsen
Cover design © 2010 by Lyle Mortimer
Edited and typeset by Heidi Doxey

Printed in the United States of America

10 9 8 7 6 5 4 3 2 1

Printed on acid-free paper

DEDICATION

For Steve—thank you for holding my hand
through the good times and bad.

And for all those who have suffered a loss.
I hope this book will help you see the
sunshine again on your cloudy day.

Contents

Acknowledgments

There are many people I want to thank who helped make this book possible. My husband, Steve, encouraged me every step of the way. My doctor, Lawrence Warner, and his kind office staff answered so many questions. Several people answered surveys and provided wonderful insight into how this trial affects each person differently. I have used many quotes from others, but changed the names to protect privacy throughout the book.

I would like to thank Janet Cox, Barbara Bodily, Shelly Olivier, Patrick and Necia Jolley, Karma Nalder, Jennifer Vest, Elise Catmull, Casey Mickelsen, Andrea Shaffer, Nichole Giles, Brittany Maxfield, Racquel Hutchings, Jen Tanner, Bret Butler, Ali Cross, Preston Farr, Andrea Jolley, Sarah Winn, Stephanie Johnson, Deana Edmondson, Stacie Henrie, and Lori Whiting.

I'm so grateful to my wonderful critique group, Cindy Beck, Connie Hall, and Nichole Giles. Thank you to the amazing people at Cedar Fort who made this book possible.

I thank my Heavenly Father every day for my beautiful children and what they teach me.

FOREWORD

We have all witnessed the repeating pattern of life, which begins with birth and ends with death, and we view this as natural and normal. But death before birth . . . well, that does not seem to fit our understanding of that plan.

All around us we observe the joy in the faces of parents with their young children. We often miss, however, the pain and hurt of lost pregnancies that those parents and others may have experienced as well.

As a practicing obstetrician for thirty-five years, I have too many times been the one who has diagnosed a failed pregnancy and had to break the news to the expectant couple that they are not going to have a child after all.

An early pregnancy loss is a very common event in nature, and a stillbirth later in pregnancy is not a rare occurrence. The emotional and physical impact on both the expectant mother and father can be easily misunderstood, underestimated, or even trivialized. A miscarriage is, in fact, a very significant and true personal loss.

Rachelle Christensen, the author of this book, has experienced the emotional devastation of two early miscarriages as well as the overwhelming joy of giving birth to beautiful, healthy children. She has successfully captured and expressed the emotions of pregnancy loss in this book, and with great empathy has set forth thoughtful and helpful advice that will benefit those in such a situation. Not only has she expressed the feelings of a mother who has experienced great loss first-hand, but also reaches out to those close to the event, including spouses, family, and friends. She shares her personal witness of the sustaining spiritual strength that she derives from her understanding and testimony of our Heavenly Father's plan of happiness and from her deep personal faith.

As you read this book, you will come to realize that you are not alone in your sorrow, and will feel added strength to endure and optimism and hope that you will recover physically, emotionally, and spiritually.

—W. Lawrence Warner, MD

INTRODUCTION

When I discovered I would become a mother, I never imagined anything would go wrong. My husband and I were overjoyed and excited to be pregnant with our first baby. We had been married for almost two years and felt ready to start a family, so we immediately began preparing for the day when we could bring our baby home.

It was an exciting time. Each day I awoke with a smile, thinking about the new life within me. I immersed myself in baby books, magazines, and any information I could find about pregnancy and becoming a mother.

About six weeks into my pregnancy, I was overcome with fear and anxiety that something was wrong with my baby. I began crying uncontrollably. My husband was concerned for me and asked me why I felt that way. I told him, "I don't know. Maybe I'm just emotional, but I'm afraid that something will go wrong with my pregnancy."

He gave me a priesthood blessing to overcome feelings of doubt and depression, and I felt at peace. I went to my first doctor appointment for my ten-week check-up and was told that everything looked good. My uterus was an appropriate size and I was in good health.

Over the next few days, I felt better and was once again excited about my pregnancy. We went shopping for a few maternity clothes. It was so fun to try on the little pregnancy pillow to see how I would look at five months pregnant. I thought back to all the Young Women lessons I had heard about the joys of motherhood and the sacred and special blessings we as women are given to be mothers. My joy was full.

When I was about eleven weeks into my pregnancy, I began spotting. I called my doctor's office, and the nurses reassured me this was common for a lot of women. After it continued for a few days, I insisted on seeing the doctor.

I prayed constantly that all would be well, but I was worried. At the appointment, my doctor tried for several minutes to find the heartbeat using the Doppler instrument. When he couldn't hear anything, he explained that sometimes it's hard to find the heartbeat in the first trimester of pregnancy. He sent us over to the hospital for an ultrasound.

I was nervous as we were admitted to the ultrasound room. The radiologist worked quietly and passed the ultrasound transducer over my abdomen. He kept looking at the fuzzy black and white images with a furrowed brow. Then he asked me, "Have you been on any fertility drugs?"

Surprised, I said, "No, this was our first try at getting pregnant."

He nodded his head and continued looking at the screen.

My husband and I watched anxiously as the radiologist enlarged the picture on the screen and three small sacs came into view.

"Is that triplets?" I asked in disbelief. He only nodded, and then I observed him make a small X in each of the three sacs. My heart sank as I watched him silently working. He didn't offer any explanation, and I was too afraid to ask. All I could do was stare at the screen with the three X marks. I wondered if he was going to wait for our doctor to give us "the news." My fears were confirmed when he finished the ultrasound and told us he would have some pictures for us to take back to our doctor in a few minutes.

I knew something was very wrong with my pregnancy. I had three sacs in my uterus but had heard no heartbeat. Still, because the radiologist had said nothing, I held on to some insane shred of hope.

My husband and I returned to our doctor's office with pictures of our ultrasound. The doctor looked them over and said, "I'm very sorry, but there was no heartbeat evident and no sign of a developing baby."

He explained that I had been pregnant with triplets, but they looked to be possibly three separate blighted ova, a pregnancy failure that had occurred so early, no clearly defined fetal tissue had formed. He explained that sometimes a pregnancy ceases to develop several weeks before the uterus actually "miscarries."

The doctor said that the gestational age looked to be about five or six weeks, which is too early to see a heartbeat. He asked that they draw my blood at that time and then again in two days to check if the HCG or pregnancy hormones in my blood were dropping. This is how we would know for sure that I would miscarry because in a viable pregnancy the HCG levels double every two days.

He offered his condolences and told me to go home, rest, and try to deal with the loss of our pregnancy. I didn't receive any instruction as to what I could do to ease the process, just a warning that if the bleeding became too heavy I should head to the emergency room.

When my husband and I returned home, I didn't want to believe I was going to have a miscarriage. Somewhere in my mind, I argued that because I had not yet lost the pregnancy, there was still a chance my babies could survive. I prayed that things would look normal with my blood tests—that maybe something was off with my cycle and I wasn't as far along as we thought. In the back of my mind, I think I knew the truth but I didn't want to let go of hope.

I thought about all the family members who knew of our pregnancy and how excited we had been to make that announcement when I was about nine weeks along. How would we tell everyone we were no longer going to have a baby?

It was difficult for me to sort out my feelings. For the past eleven weeks, I had been on an emotional high, preparing to be a mother. It was hard to believe that it wasn't going to happen. Physically, I felt fine and kept hoping some miracle would take place. At the same time, I could hardly believe I had been pregnant with triplets. What an amazing event! We couldn't help but talk about what it would have been like to have three babies at once. My husband was still in college, and I had recently graduated. We told ourselves we could never have afforded three babies at once in our little trailer home, but this make-believe consolation didn't offer any comfort.

After a few days, I experienced intense pain and cramping. I was bleeding heavily and couldn't stop dry-heaving from the pain. I called my husband at work and told him I needed help. He rushed home and took me to the emergency room.

That was the worst day of my life. I felt lost. While I waited in the emergency room, my body writhed with pain, which was all the more devastating because there would be no reward for any of it—only sorrow.

After I was treated, we returned to our empty home. We were devastated. I spent an entire day lying on the couch crying and asking the Lord why He let this happen. My husband was deeply saddened by our loss. He worried for me with the pain I had gone through and the recovery ahead. After months of pure joy and excitement, we were now left with emptiness. We were in a young married student ward where almost every couple had children. I didn't know anyone who had experienced a miscarriage, and I had never expected to go through this trial.

All the tears I cried could not wash away the insurmountable level of grief surrounding me. I received a priesthood blessing, but this did not completely take away my sorrow.

As I went through the grieving process, I was left with many unanswered questions. I wondered what had happened to my babies. Were they developed enough to house a spirit? I was told by many people that I would have a celestial baby to raise in the hereafter, but that didn't bring me comfort because I couldn't find Church doctrine to support the claim.

A year after that experience, I wrote the following in my journal: "I felt prompted to write about how to deal with miscarriage because maybe I could help someone in need." At the time I didn't know that the "someone" would be me. The Lord was already preparing a way for me to face another challenge in my life.

Ten months later I wrote: "The temple holds such a beautiful and peaceful feeling. It brings life into perspective. All I want is to have a baby. I know the Lord will bless us soon."

After my miscarriage, people gave me all sorts of advice, and although they meant well, much of it was misinformed. I struggled with going to church because it seemed there was always someone asking, "When are you going to have kids?" or offering suggestions and distorted doctrine. I searched for answers to my questions, received priesthood blessings, and met with my bishop to help me through the grieving process.

My husband and I were married for nearly five years before we were able to have our first baby. In that time I experienced two miscarriages and problems with infertility. Finally, our first daughter was born on a beautiful April day nearly three years after my first miscarriage. Two years later in August, we were blessed with another beautiful daughter, and three years later, a son. Though nothing brings me more joy today than my children, I still remember the deep sense of longing and loss I felt when I had no children.

This is why I have written this book. I hope the information and experiences I have gathered from many books, doctors, and people who have experienced a miscarriage, stillbirth, or infertility will help you through your time of sadness. I realize there are many who have suffered greater tribulations than I have experienced. For this reason, I have studied diligently to uncover truths that I hope will also help you through your trials.

I have a strong testimony of the gospel of Jesus Christ, and I know my Heavenly Father has a plan for me and for each of you. He loves us and He will never leave us, if we will but come unto Him.

chapter 1

WHAT IS a
MISCARRIAGE?

Miscarriage is medically defined as a "spontaneous abortion" of the fetus before twenty weeks of gestation (as opposed to a "therapeutic abortion," which is considered when a pregnancy threatens maternal life). The term *spontaneous abortion* often carries a negative connotation, but if you read or hear about spontaneous abortions, this actually refers to miscarriages.

One in three hundred couples will have three or more consecutive miscarriages, and one in four pregnancies ends in miscarriage. This means that in their lifetime almost all people will know someone who has experienced this trial, yet few women talk about their losses openly. Millions of people will be affected by the loss miscarriage brings. You are not alone.

Most miscarriages occur in the first thirteen weeks, or first trimester, of pregnancy. Some miscarriages occur before a woman misses her menstrual period or is even aware she is pregnant. This may be the body's way of ending a pregnancy in which the fetus was not growing normally and would not have been able to survive.

The cause of miscarriage is often unknown, but there are some known factors that could contribute to miscarriage. These include fertilization late after ovulation, low or high levels of thyroid hormone, uncontrolled diabetes, uterine abnormalities, certain medications, caffeine consumption, and exposure to radiation or toxic agents. Hormone imbalance and the body's inability to produce enough of certain hormones, such as progesterone, can cause miscarriage. Immune system problems, such as being Rh-negative, can cause miscarriage and other difficulties with pregnancy. Most of these issues are treatable. For example, women who are Rh-negative can receive a shot called Rhogam to keep their immune systems from attacking their babies' red blood cells. Women low in the hormone progesterone can take a pill, usually for the first trimester, to support the baby.

In some cases there are problems with the uterus or the cervix that can lead to miscarriage, usually in the second trimester (14–28 weeks) of pregnancy. Some women have abnormally shaped uteruses, which make pregnancy difficult. Other women have incompetent cervixes that begin to widen and open early, in the middle part of pregnancy. This often occurs without any signs of labor, and the fetus is too young to survive.

Chromosomal abnormalities are the most common causes of miscarriage and are found in more than half of miscarriages occurring in the first thirteen weeks. Miscarriages apparently eliminate about 95 percent of fertilized eggs or embryos with genetic problems—our body's natural way of ending a pregnancy in which the child would be unable to survive. The chromosomes in the nucleus of both the egg and sperm need to join into twenty-three pairs for a total of forty-six chromosomes. Sometimes the pairing of these chromosomes doesn't happen correctly, and that creates an unstable embryo.

Miscarriages of this type usually occur before the woman even knows she is pregnant. Most chromosomal abnormalities happen by chance, have nothing to do with the parents, and are unlikely to recur. If three or more miscarriages have occurred, however, couples are advised to seek medical evaluation to identify a specific cause, if possible.

TYPES OF MISCARRIAGE

- A **blighted ovum** is a miscarriage that has occurred so early, no clearly defined fetal tissue has formed.
- A **threatened miscarriage** occurs when bleeding or cramping begins and yet the pregnancy is still viable at the time of evaluation.
- An **inevitable miscarriage** refers to bleeding and cramping during the early stages of pregnancy and usually indicates that the cervix is opening.
- An **incomplete miscarriage** happens when the woman's body has not completely expelled all the elements of the pregnancy.
- A **missed miscarriage** occurs when the pregnancy has stopped developing but the body has not discharged the fetus, the placenta, or other elements of the pregnancy.
- **Recurrent miscarriage** is a term used when a woman miscarries three or more consecutive times.
- **Ectopic pregnancy** is another factor in the loss of pregnancy. This occurs when the fertilized egg doesn't reach the uterus. It may grow in the fallopian tube or attach to an ovary or another organ in the abdomen. Almost all ectopic pregnancies occur in the fallopian tube. The tube is narrow and its wall are thin, so the pregnancy can grow to only about the size of a walnut before the tube bursts. These problems can occur any time in the first three months of pregnancy. An ectopic pregnancy can be very dangerous for a mother because the fallopian tube may burst and cause severe bleeding in the abdomen or even death. Once diagnosed, tubal pregnancy must be treated promptly.
- **Molar pregnancy** is a rare disease of pregnancy also called gestational trophoblastic disease (GTD), or simply a mole. It results in the growth of abnormal tissue, not an embryo. Molar pregnancy occurs in 1 of every 1,500–2,000 pregnancies.

Dispelling the Miscarriage Myths

"It's my fault my baby died." Many women believe they are responsible for their miscarriages because they fell down or had some other minor accident, were exposed to something harmful, or even overworked themselves. The truth is that a miscarriage is rarely related to anything the mother did. In most cases, it occurs because of chromosomal abnormalities that are out of our control.

"If I begin spotting, I will have a miscarriage." Many women have spotting or bleeding during the early stages of pregnancy. Spotting is usually not a cause for alarm unless it continues and increases or is accompanied by cramping. Even though spotting is fairly common, it is okay to call or visit your doctor with questions, and I would recommend doing so for your own peace of mind.

"If I have a miscarriage, I will never be able to have a successful pregnancy." Even though miscarriages are common, less than 1 percent of all couples experience three or more miscarriages, and many of those who do still go on to have children. Having a miscarriage doesn't automatically exclude you from successful child-bearing. Talk to your doctor about when it's safe for you to try again. Most women who have miscarried go on to have successful pregnancies.

"A miscarriage always happens because of problems with the woman's body." This is not true. Most miscarriages are caused by chromosomal abnormalities that can be linked back to either the man or the woman. In the event of recurrent miscarriages, testing can be done to discover the source of the problem. Some conditions found in both the man and the woman can affect pregnancy loss.

Stillbirth

A small fraction of miscarriages, less than 1 percent, are called stillbirths because they occur after twenty weeks of gestation. A stillbirth or intrauterine death may occur prior to labor or during the labor and delivery process. The cause of about one-third of all stillbirths remains unknown, but the most common known causes of stillbirth include the following:

Placental abruption: The premature separation of the placenta from the uterine wall. There is an increased chance of this occurring in pregnant women who have high blood pressure or preeclampsia (toxemia). Sometimes abnormal placental development and function may result in an insufficient amount of oxygen and nutrients getting to the baby, and this may result in death.

Birth Defects: Chromosomal abnormalities account for 5–10 percent of all stillborn babies. Sometimes a baby has structural malformations that are not caused by chromosomal abnormalities, but can result from genetic, environmental, or unknown causes.

Growth Restriction: Babies who are small or not growing at an appropriate rate are at risk of death from asphyxia (lack of oxygen) both before labor or during the birth process. Even if asphyxia does not occur, these babies can also die from other unknown causes.

Infection: Bacterial or viral infections can cause fetal deaths. These infections usually go unnoticed by the mother and may not be diagnosed until they cause serious complications.

Other possible causes of stillbirth include umbilical cord accidents, trauma, maternal diabetes, high blood pressure, and postdate pregnancy (a pregnancy that lasts longer than forty-two weeks).

The most common symptom of stillbirth is loss of movement in the baby. The diagnosis is confirmed by ultrasound when no fetal heart motion is detected. Stillbirth is not rare, and it may affect anyone. There is no way to predict if stillbirth will happen or who will experience it, as this occurs in families of all races, regions, and income levels.

Because stillbirth is closely related to miscarriage, I have tried to provide information throughout this book to help with both situations but for simplicity's sake I will usually refer to the event as miscarriage.

FACTS ON INFERTILITY

It is common for normal, healthy couples to take several months to conceive. Most doctors will recommend that you try to get pregnant for at least six months before attempting to diagnose or treat infertility problems. The medical definition of infertility is the failure to become pregnant after one year of trying. There are such a wide range of problems that contribute to infertility that it is difficult to diagnose. It often takes much more time to diagnose and treat than we would like. It may be helpful to seek out a specialist in infertility who will evaluate both the husband and the wife to find the source of the problem, if possible.

chapter 2

LDS Doctrine on Miscarriage and Stillbirth

Why? Why? Why?

The most common question anyone will ask when facing a miscarriage, a stillbirth, or infertility is "Why? Why did this happen to me?" From my own experiences, I was told, "There is no reason. Sadly, there is not enough information—we don't know why." This was probably the most frustrating part for me because I desperately wanted to know why.

I still don't have all the specific answers I once sought, but I have grown spiritually and I feel at peace with my Heavenly Father's plan. I now understand fully that there was a reason I suffered through my miscarriages—and there was more than one reason. I had to go through this trial for my own personal growth and to help others who experienced miscarriages. I know my Heavenly Father and Jesus Christ have provided the most perfect plan for me to learn, and my trials are part of what makes the plan divine.

If someone had asked me during those years of suffering and wanting a child if I would ever look back and say that I was glad I had experienced these things, I would have said, "Absolutely not!"

But now I realize that even though those experiences were painful and I hated all the disappointment and discouragement, they were also necessary. As we read in Doctrine and Covenants, "all these things shall give thee experience, and shall be for thy good" (122: 7). I am grateful for what I have learned from the trials I experienced. I am a different and better person because of my trials.

LDS Doctrine

I have come across several "versions" of what happens to the spirit involved with a miscarriage or stillbirth, but there is some specific church doctrine available on these subjects. The Church Handbook of Instructions says:

> Grieving parents whose child dies before birth should be given emotional and spiritual support. Temple ordinances are not performed for stillborn children. However, this does not deny the possibility that a stillborn child may be part of the family in the eternities. Parents are encouraged to trust the Lord to resolve such cases in the way He knows is best. The family may record the name of a stillborn child on the family group record followed by the word "stillborn" in parentheses. Memorial or grave-side services may be held as determined by the parents.
>
> It is a fact that a child has life before birth. However, there is no direct revelation on when the spirit enters the body.[1]

Elder Bruce R. McConkie explained: "These are matters not clearly answered in the revelation so far available for the guidance of the saints in this dispensation. No doubt such things were plainly set forth in those past dispensations when more of the doctrines of salvation were known and taught than have been revealed so far to us."[2]

In the September 1987 *Ensign*, Val D. Greenwood answered this question: "Can we put the names of our miscarried or stillborn children on our family group records? Will these children belong to us in the hereafter?" He answered,

> Church policy does permit a family to record stillborn children on their family group record if they wish to do so.... Miscarriages, however, are not normally recorded. The line between a miscarriage and a stillbirth is not clear-cut, and sometimes there is a question as to

whether the fetus was viable. In this case, the decision to record or not to record the name on the family records is up to the family.

Elder Joseph Fielding Smith wrote, "there is no information given by revelation in regard to the status of stillborn children. However, I will express my personal opinion that we should have hope that these little ones will receive a resurrection and then belong to us."

Though our knowledge of the plan of salvation does not explain why miscarriages and stillbirths take place, nor what the eternal result will be, we can know with confidence that God, who is the father of all spirits, is merciful and just. We can know also that there is hope. Worthy parents can trust in him and know that they and all his spirit children will—one way or another—receive a just reward for their efforts and sacrifice, perhaps in ways that we do not presently comprehend.[3]

WHERE IS MY BABY?

Almost everyone I interviewed who had experienced a miscarriage wanted to know why it had happened. Was Heavenly Father just testing them or was it a health-related problem? They wanted to know where their baby went and if they would in fact have another chance to raise that spirit on earth or in heaven.

A very wise person told me that we need to realize the world is not perfect. In fact, it is full of imperfections. When Adam fell, the world fell also, and it is currently in a telestial state. As a natural result, tragic things happen in our fallen, mortal, earthly condition. However, Heavenly Father did create a plan of happiness for us, and Jesus Christ created the world to move in harmony with that plan.

Nature is in harmony with the plan and as a result, there are many imperfect events in nature, including miscarriage, stillbirth, and infertility. These are not errors in our Father's plan, but flaws in our imperfect world. Just as many people die from sickness and experience pain because of the diseases that abound in our imperfect world, so will many women suffer from miscarriage, stillbirth, and infertility. It helps to understand that Heavenly Father is not punishing us; He allows us to experience the consequences of our imperfect world so that we might grow and become the people He would have us be.

Though these words are not the answer most of us want to hear, we will understand everything in due time. The Lord may see fit to reveal to you during your lifetime the reasons this happened. Or you may find out after this life, when so many of our questions will be answered by the greatest teacher of all time.

One of my seminary teachers taught a lesson I still recall. He drew a circle on the board and inside it he wrote, "Things we need to know." Then he drew another circle around it and wrote, "Things we want to know." Then he wrote outside of both circles, "Things that we will know." This represents the stages of our life. There is a vast amount of doctrine we should study and learn while on this earth, yet no matter how much we study we will still have some unanswered questions that must wait until after we pass through the veil and our former state is restored.

Sometimes medical doctors can find physical evidence as to why a miscarriage or stillbirth occurred, but generally we are left with unanswered questions. This carries over to the spiritual state of the baby as well. I think the hardest part about dealing with a miscarriage or stillbirth is all the unknowns—the inability to rely on anything concrete to help us through this ordeal. If we could just make sense of our situations, it would be easier to make our way through the grieving process.

Through writing this book, I feel the Lord has blessed me all over again with a deeper understanding of why my miscarriages happened. I have learned so much through my research, surveys, and the comments I gathered from others. I know I do not fully understand the imperfect world we live in, but I also know that if I live righteously I will be able to witness the perfection of all things.

Heavenly Father does provide each of us with personal inspiration. He can help us make sense of our situations and provide personal revelation to guide us through our trials. But He will determine what to reveal, how to reveal it to us, and, most important, when this revelation will come. This doesn't mean that just because we are righteous we'll know things He hasn't yet seen fit to reveal, but it does mean that it is okay to pray for understanding and to have a belief about what happened to your baby.

Ellen shared her experience:

I believe every mother must come to her own decision, through prayer and priesthood direction if necessary, as to the fate of her child. Will that child be waiting in the afterlife, as some may suggest, or will that child have another chance to gain a body, as others will tell you? I believe the answer varies in many cases and can only be found through prayer. I believe I received confirmation that the child I lost was the child I gave birth to less than ten months later. I do not believe her spirit had entered her body at the time of the miscarriage. This confirmation brought me much peace, even before I knew I was expecting again. That said, when I die, if there is another child waiting for me, that is just fine with me. I will accept that child with open arms. I'm just not going to count on it.

A bishop shared his thoughts: "Several questions arise, . . . [including] did the spirit ever enter the body? If it did, then obviously parents who live worthily will have the opportunity to raise that child during the Millennium. If it did not, then that spirit would be given an opportunity to be born again."

We are all given the opportunity to receive revelation from our Father in Heaven. After searching the doctrine available to you, I suggest you seek the Lord in faith to help you understand your trials and find purpose in your suffering. "He that diligently seeketh shall find; and the mysteries of God shall be unfolded unto them, by the power of the Holy Ghost" (1 Nephi 10:19).

FINDING SOLACE IN THE SCRIPTURES

I love to hold my scriptures and touch their fine pages. At times I can feel the presence of the Spirit so powerfully radiating from within those pages. The scriptures are a direct channel or link to our Heavenly Father and all that He has revealed to help us understand our sojourn on earth. Following are some of the verses that have helped me.

This first scripture reminds us that one day we will understand all that God has not yet revealed to us. In the Book of Mormon, Nephi exclaimed, "O how great the plan of our God! For on the other hand, the paradise of God must deliver up the spirits of the righteous, and the grave deliver up the body of the righteous; and the spirit and the body is restored to itself again, and all men become incorruptible, and immortal, and they are living souls, having a perfect knowledge like unto us in the flesh, save it be that our knowledge shall be perfect" (2 Nephi 9:13).

In the Bible, Job is a symbol of suffering and trials. He lost his entire family and even his existence seemed damned, but Job was reminded that there is a reason for everything and that God is greater than anything we can comprehend. In Job 37 we read of God's perfect knowledge and plan for all things. "Hearken unto this, O Job: stand still, and consider the wondrous works of God. . . . Dost thou know the balancings of the clouds, the wondrous works of him which is perfect in knowledge?" (14–15). And Job 36:4 reiterates a witness of His omniscience. "For truly my words shall not be false: he that is perfect in knowledge is with thee."

I asked many people what their favorite comforting scriptures were and was grateful to discover more meaning in some of the scriptures that were already familiar to me. I found that when I studied the scriptures with a specific prayer in my heart, I noticed things I had previously missed.

One scripture that has offered comfort to many is found in Matthew 11. "Come unto me, all ye that labour and are heavy laden, and I will give you rest. Take my yoke upon you, and learn of me; for I am meek and lowly in heart: and ye shall find rest unto your souls. For my yoke is easy, and my burden is light" (28–30).

An LDS Doctor's Thoughts

My current obstetrician has offered wonderful insights to help me understand the trials I went through before I had children. He said we need to remember that we are all Heavenly Father's children. Heavenly Father loves us, and He has designed for us the plan of happiness, not the plan of misery. This includes a veil over our memory of the premortal world. Even though we don't fully understand all its details, this doesn't diminish the greatness of our Father's plan for us. My obstetrician reminded me "not to attempt to expound on what the Lord has not yet revealed to us."

Instead we need to rely on our understanding of the Creation and the Fall of Adam. Because of imperfections, an estimated 35–45 percent of conceptions fail. Because of imperfections, tragedy happens all around us each day. The horrible hurricane Katrina of 2005 destroyed homes and families and took many lives. The earthquake in Haiti in 2010 killed thousands. Did the Lord cause this hurricane or this earthquake? No, but He allowed the events to happen because we live in an imperfect world.

We understand that every spirit who kept its first estate is entitled to come to earth and experience both birth—to gain a physical body—and death—in order to return to God. Brigham Young suggested that the spirit entered the body or there was a quickening of the spirit when the woman first felt the baby move inside her.[4] But now we can detect life through the evidence of a beating heart from the very first weeks of pregnancy. The way we perceive something and the reality of a situation may be two different things.

Notes

1. Church Handbook of Instructions, 185.
2. Bruce R. McConkie, *Mormon Doctrine*, 2nd ed. (Salt Lake City: Bookcraft, 1979), 674.
3. Val D. Greenwood, "I Have a Question," *Ensign*, Sept. 1987, 27; quoting *Doctrines of Salvation*, 2:280.
4. Ibid., quoting *Journal of Discourses*, 17:143.

chapter 3

Coping

Emotionally

As Latter-day Saints, our goals are to live virtuously, marry in the temple, keep the commandments, and raise righteous families. We have been commanded to "multiply and replenish the earth." After working diligently to choose the right, we find ourselves on the path—that strait and narrow yet elusive path we have sought so fervently. We are overwhelmed with joy as we anticipate the promise of so many blessings that will soon be ours when we begin a family. Then suddenly, hopes are shattered. When a miscarriage happens, the blessing of having that sweet baby is ripped from our arms, and it is so hard not to question why this is happening to us.

But I want to share that I believe He hears us. One of Hilary Weeks' songs says, "He hears me, when I'm crying in the night. He hears me, when my soul longs to fight. 'til the morning will come and the light of the dawn reassures, He hears me."[1]

Did you know the Savior's Atonement covers all of our suffering? His suffering in Gethsemane was not just for our sins, but for all the negative emotions we experience. He knows and feels our anguish, our sadness, our grief. I heard a sister in my ward bear her testimony about the Atonement and how it encompasses every human emotion, and I realized I had never considered the Atonement in that specific way. I had always thought of the Atonement as my tool for repentance since I knew Jesus Christ had suffered for all of our sins. But He suffered for me, even in my anguish and despair as I struggled to have a child. I knew He understood our feelings, but I hadn't realized that the power of the Atonement is how He understands every part of what we suffer.

I encourage you to grasp onto the Atonement, this priceless gift our Savior has given to us. Rely on Him and allow Him to guide you through your sorrows. Do as Proverbs 3:5 instructs: "Trust in the Lord with all thine heart; and lean not unto thine own understanding."

The Holy Ghost is our Comforter, a special gift bestowed upon every member of the Church. He is there to guide, protect, and comfort us. In John 14:16, Jesus explained to the disciples that Heavenly Father would provide another source of comfort to them when He left the earth. "And I will pray the Father, and he shall give you another Comforter, that he may abide with you for ever."

We teach our children from the earliest ages about the Comforter and help them to understand that the Holy Ghost is here to help each of us throughout our lives. Sometimes we forget that this remains true for us as adults. The Comforter is such a unique and wonderful gift, and if we seek His presence and help, we can feel His comforting power envelop us and cushion us against life's deepest trials.

When I first became pregnant, I excitedly filled out all the little cards for free information and baby magazine subscriptions. I remember after my miscarriage how hard it was to get the mail and see the baby magazines that kept coming. Even several months later, I would think I was getting over it but would go to the mailbox and find a little pamphlet with information about my third trimester or something similar. I would bite my lip all the way home and try not to cry. It was especially hard after I had passed my due date and I received "Congratulations!" postcards in the mail from baby companies. I wanted a baby so badly, and everywhere I turned there were reminders that I didn't have a baby and had no hope of one yet.

One of my friends suggested: "Let yourself mourn, it helps. I tried to be strong and just get over it. That doesn't work. You have to mourn, talk about it, read about it. Do things to celebrate what you do have. Do not neglect your family (including your other children and your husband)."

I wish I could promise you that you will feel better by a certain time, but we are all different. Some of us will mourn for longer periods of time than others. Some of us will try to put off experiencing our grief and then have it overcome us later. There are many ways to deal with grief. I think in the situation of a miscarriage or stillbirth, it is important to recognize there will be grief and a period of mourning.

I'm thankful to Hailey for allowing me to include her story.

> At our twenty-week ultrasound, we found out that our baby had passed away about three weeks earlier. Because I was far enough along in my pregnancy, I had to be induced into labor. I delivered our baby girl the next day. She weighed four ounces and was eight inches long. We gave her a name, but chose not to have a funeral service. . . .
>
> It's normal to experience all the stages of grief. Grieving and healing take time and are unique to each individual. Don't berate yourself for what you're feeling—days, weeks, even months after your experience. Time really is a great healer, but the amount of time is different for everyone. With difficult trials come blessings of compensation. If we look for them and remember to trust in the Lord, even the toughest of situations can become a chance for spiritual growth, marital closeness, and compassion.

It may help to know that you are not alone. Although you may be unaware, there are women all around you who have suffered from miscarriage. Sometimes if we reach out to others, they can bridge the gap and help us through our sorrows. Seek help from Heavenly Father and by receiving priesthood blessings.

Satan will be there trying to fill your heart with anger and bitterness. The saying, "Misery loves company," is all too true because Satan tempts us in our times of trials to forsake our beliefs and forget who we are. You might experience feelings of great anger and frustration at your situation, but you must not yield to Satan's temptations and forget the greatness of our Heavenly Father's plan. When you start feeling miserable, don't invite Satan's company. Instead, invite the Comforter to help you. Invite your friends and family to support you in your times of need.

In Alma 7:12, we read that Christ suffered so "that he may know according to the flesh how to succor his people according to their infirmities" (see also v. 11). We must keep perspective and seek out the unconditional love our Savior is willing to give us. The Savior is omniscient; we must trust Him and have faith that He knows how to comfort us.

Don't Talk to Me! Everything Hurts!

Abraham Lincoln said, "If you look for the bad in mankind expecting to find it, you surely will."[2] How can we overcome being offended and oversensitive? Some of you may wonder why you should even have to worry about such a thing when you have so many other thoughts and feelings you are trying to sort through. I think it is best to be prepared and know that you will hear some comments that may offend you *if* you let them.

Imagine a large window in a spacious home. The weather outside is changing to autumn. The leaves on the tree are starting to change colors and fall to the ground. The wind is rustling the leaves, and bits of orange and brown are swirling about on the green grass. Two people can look out the same window and see two completely different things.

People who love autumn will feel excitement when they look out the window. They love the chill in the air. They look forward to family gatherings and snowy mountains. They are grateful for the beauty that surrounds them. Others, however, may scowl and grumble about the coming cold weather, the leaves to be raked, the wood to be hauled for fires, and the bitter winter they will have to endure. The happiness in our lives is usually determined by our perspective.

Interacting with others is often difficult during a grieving period. So what should we say when someone asks a personal question about our miscarriage? Put things into perspective. The best advice I ever heard was to answer, "Why do you ask?" With this simple response, we can avoid becoming angry and hurt and hopefully uncover the reason the person is asking. This can apply to any situation in life because we will all probably have to answer curious, yet uncomfortable questions from well-meaning individuals.

By turning the question around, we can alert the person in a tactful way that they have asked something personal. If they choose to continue the thread of questioning or explain why they are asking, we will usually discover they are asking because they sincerely care and not because they intend to offend.

We can clear the fog from our windows and appreciate other people's concern for us if we remember how much the Savior loves us and realize that most people are trying to be like Him. No matter what the circumstance, there is always the potential for a kind response. Part of learning charity is not being easily offended and also assuming the best in every situation.

In order to overcome offense, we have to put ourselves in others' shoes. I know that is exactly what we wish *they* would do for *us*, but if we will really think about how hard it is for people to know what to say to someone experiencing a loss, perhaps we can find their sincere concern under the layers of hurtful questions and comments. It is better to remember to be forgiving and be grateful that we have learned how to respond to someone in need so that we won't make the same mistakes.

The afflicted can make it easier for others to comfort them. I reminded myself over and over again not to be offended. It helped me to try to see others as Christ saw them and then recognize that He was trying to help me through others. People are not perfect and neither am I, but Christ is perfect and so is our Heavenly Father's plan. My prayer often has been to ask Heavenly Father to help me know people as Christ knows them.

Christ is perfect because He has experienced and understands all human emotions. Christ could love His enemies because He could see inside their hearts and see why they were acting in certain ways. He could truly love His enemies because He knew them. Someone I admire pointed out to me that it is very easy to love someone who loves you back, but what makes us Christlike is to love those who don't love us.

Heavenly Father's plan teaches us how to love, and we are given experiences daily that allow us to choose to love someone and demonstrate that love in how we react to what they say or do.

It is very hard not to take offense when we are feeling vulnerable. We feel so hurt and raw that it is painful whenever someone comes close to our wounds. One of my favorite quotes is from Eleanor Roosevelt. She said, "No one can make you feel inferior without your consent."[3]

In preparation for writing this book, I created several different surveys that many people responded to. One question I asked was, "If there was one thing you wish you could tell someone who has just experienced any of these problems [miscarriage, stillbirth, or infertility], what would it be?"

A friend responded,

> People will say dumb, hurtful, and inconsiderate things. It's a given—they will. But they don't say them to be dumb, hurtful, and inconsiderate. They say them because they don't know what else to say. They say them out of love. It does no good to hold grudges and be angry over something someone said. They probably didn't mean to hurt you, but rather were trying to comfort you. My example—an older sister at church patted me on the back and said, "You're young. You'll be able to have another baby." I went home bawling. I didn't want another baby—I wanted THAT baby! Looking back, maybe she lost a child when she was too old to try again. I'm sure she was trying to lend comfort, but at the time I was furious and hurt.

Another response I received was a wonderful reminder of how most people would never dream of intentionally hurting us. It's all about how we view the situation.

> Sometimes people who are struggling with infertility and miscarriage are offended when others talk about their children or announce new pregnancies. Rather than feeling that you have a right to be angry at them, you should consider this question: Do you think people should pretend their children and babies do not exist because you do not have one?
>
> We will not all have the same things in this world. Yes, it may be painful to hear others talk, but instead of retreating into your shell, spin things around and think, "How does my Savior see this person?" Of course the Savior loves all children, and I'm sure He would be happy to see that people's lives revolve around their children. He would also

notice you and hope you are learning as much as you can, because if you are righteous, you will be a parent someday. It may not be in this life, but you will be granted all the righteous desires of your heart in the eternities.

Women who have experienced a miscarriage, stillbirth, or problems with infertility sometimes feel angry when they overhear parents complaining about their children. As I mentioned before, if you look for reasons to feel bitter or angry, I'm sure you will find them. However, if you've suffered from the trial of losing a baby, this does not mean you will be a perfect parent. I do believe that couples who have traveled a long and difficult road to become parents may seem to appreciate their children more, but even they may still have bad days, and yes, even they may sometimes complain. No one on this earth is perfect. If I may, I would suggest that you not be angry with other people because they have kids and occasionally complain about them. It certainly doesn't mean they don't love their children; it just means the parents are human.

Lori experienced recurrent miscarriages and shared how she felt:

> When I was sad and hurting because the children I longed for had not yet come into my life, I used to be sure I would be such a better mom than most of the moms I saw. And I would never complain about my children. But now that my children are here and I sometimes get swept up in the busy-ness of life, I surprise myself from time to time by the thoughtless things I say. In that moment of frustration or exhaustion, I might say something unkind about my child.
>
> I'm sorry when I say those things because I love my children with all my heart and I am so grateful they finally came into my life. But the truth is, sometimes life gets away from us, and these little people do complicate things.
>
> If you are one whose arms are still empty, I understand how you may sometimes find yourself feeling hurt by the thoughtless comments other moms might say about their children. I hope you can find it in your heart to forgive them because they are just human and are trying to do their best day by day.

Doctrine and Covenants 68:6 is a good reminder of how to deal with unpleasant situations: "Wherefore, be of good cheer, and do not fear, for I the Lord am with you, and will stand by you."

A RIGHT TO GRIEVE AND OVERCOMING GRIEF

Almost two years after my first miscarriage, and after dealing with infertility issues, I became pregnant again, but then we experienced our second miscarriage. I remember thinking during the time before this, "I could never survive going through a second miscarriage." Despite that thought, I felt sustained by my Savior and supported by my loving family.

Miscarriage statistics aren't well publicized, and most people are surprised by how common miscarriages are. Dealing with miscarriage might be much easier if a weight of silence didn't hang over the topic. If those suffering can feel comfortable with their right to grieve and gain support from others, they will weather their trials better. Without an acknowledgment that the grief of a miscarriage is real, many people may feel that they suffer alone. I think one of the most difficult aspects of a miscarriage is that there is usually no physical evidence of the loss, and so people think that a person shouldn't grieve.

Whether you were three weeks or nineteen weeks pregnant at the time of your miscarriage, you may experience a great sense of loss, and you have a right and a need to grieve. I hear so many women say, "Well, she was only six weeks along," or "I was only seven weeks along." Some people will take comfort in knowing they weren't very far into their pregnancy, but it wasn't any comfort to me when my second miscarriage happened at seven weeks. From the minute I discovered I was pregnant, I was thrilled and once again felt all the emotions of any expectant mother. For those few weeks of my pregnancy, my husband and I were so excited. Just because I was only seven weeks along when I miscarried does not mean I shouldn't have had the right to mourn my loss.

There is no medical statement that says you must be a certain number of weeks pregnant before you can mourn your loss, should you miscarry. If someone chooses to use this explanation to comfort themselves, that is fine, but I would not personally discount someone else's pregnancy loss.

Our society often fails to recognize the nature of miscarriage and its associated feelings of loss. Most people acknowledge and allow the feelings of grief that parents feel after losing an infant at a few days or a few months of age, but miscarriage is often dismissed. And the same feelings of loss that parents experience when they lose a child before birth are often considered unnecessary. I think these misconceptions come about because of ignorance. Everyone who experiences the loss of a baby, whether through miscarriage, stillbirth, or after a successful birth will experience grief, and all are entitled to their specific grieving process, regardless of society's traditions.

Trisha spoke about the difficulties of grieving alone. "I think it would have helped me a great deal to have someone besides myself recognize that my loss was similar or equal to a death and my grief was reasonable. I think if anyone had taken that attitude during my sad time, the grief I felt might have been easier to deal with, and maybe it might have passed more quickly."

One article explains, "Experts traditionally viewed pregnancy and infant loss as a transient, personal event, but we now recognize that parents often experience fetal and infant deaths, particularly those after the first trimester, as traumatic events that can trigger profound grief in the parent and sometimes lead to prolonged grief, guilt, depression, and anxiety."[4]

I want to emphasize that in the event of a miscarriage, the couple has the same right to grieve as anyone who has ever lost a loved one. During this grieving process, the woman's body is trying to readjust both physically and mentally. All the hormones that were being made for the pregnancy will suddenly stop production, and this creates a different environment in her body. It is not the woman's fault that these changes are occurring, and there is nothing that can be done to stop the miscarriage process from happening. Our bodies are miracles at work, and they know what needs to be done to ensure survival.

The emotional trauma of miscarriage may require a longer recovery time than the physical healing of the body. The bond between a mother and her baby is immediate, and the sense of loss is real, even if the pregnancy ends in the first few weeks.

As soon as a woman discovers she is pregnant, she will mark a date on her calendar. It is her due date, the day she will welcome home her newborn baby. The countdown to that date is like a thousand Christmas countdowns combined. She and her husband are busily making arrangements for this joyful baby to come into their lives.

When a miscarriage occurs, the calendar is still there, hanging on the wall. Even though we would like to stop time, the due date looms in the distance. The baby toys, sleepers, and books we bought still fill the shelves, and the afghan in progress for the baby's blessing is a reminder of the unfulfilled hopes and dreams of that little family. It is hard to understand the situation.

When I experienced my first miscarriage, I felt like a piece of my life was taken from me. Suddenly I didn't know how to be happy, when it seemed just moments before I was happier than I thought possible. With all the hopes of becoming a new mother lifting me each day, I had thought of my pregnancy and my new baby constantly. Afterward, all I could think about was the loss.

Grief can take on many forms and can be a very different experience for each person. As you are searching for answers and trying to cope with your loss, you may experience a number of different symptoms such as loss of appetite, headaches, disrupted sleep, anxiousness, or even depression.

The most severe cases of grief result from a death that is unexpected, tragic, or unexplained. Miscarriage falls into each of these categories. It is difficult to know how to deal with miscarriage because most often there is no explanation. When you break a bone, you know why it happened and how to fix it. Unfortunately, with miscarriage the meanings and remedies are not so clear-cut.

Miscarriage does represent a loss, and people do experience real grief as a result of this loss. It was so hard for me when people would just brush it off and say things like, "Oh, you'll have another one," or "My friend had four miscarriages," as if I should be comforted by the mere fact that someone had experienced more miscarriages than I.

This was a real baby, and we were planning and preparing for it, loving it and praying for it. But not everyone understood the whole gamut of emotions we faced. For many, miscarrying may not seem the same as losing a loved one, but for the mother experiencing it, that pregnancy was the beginning of the greatest love of her life.

Of course there is a difference between losing a fetus that has not even been born yet and the loss of someone already living on the earth, but in spite of the differences, the emotions experienced may be very similar in both situations. As was mentioned earlier, everyone will pass through the same stages of grief in their own unique order. The difference lies in how we move through each stage.

We are created to have continuous hope in our journey through life, so we experience some of our most profound times of sadness when those hopes are crushed. At the same time, we have been given the gift of the Holy Ghost. The Holy Ghost is our Comforter, and He plays a special role in overcoming grief. When we lose a loved one to death, a hole is created in the fabric of our lives, but the Holy Ghost can mend the hole that death leaves behind. As we rely on the Atonement and seek the Comforter, the gaping hole is mended—even those holes created by the trials of miscarriage and infertility.

Understanding grief and the specific type of grief you will feel as you pass through trials is difficult. Grieving is a very complex process, and there's not one easy answer for it. We can pray for help as we experience these emotions, and the Savior will carry us through them. As He said, "I will not leave you comfortless; I will come to you." (John 14:18).

Notes

1. Hilary Weeks, *The Collection*, compact disc, track 2: "He Hears Me," Lumen Records, 2007.
2. Abraham Lincoln, http://www.gaia.com/quotes/Abraham_Lincoln.
3. Eleanor Roosevelt, http://www.wisdomquotes.com/cat_selfrespect.html.
4. Katherine J. Gold, Vanessa K. Dalton, Thomas L. Schwenk MDs, "Hospital Care for Parents After Perinatal Death," *Obstetrics & Gynecology*, vol. 109, no. 5, May 2007.

chapter 4

COPING
PHYSICALLY

During my research, I came upon many conflicting pieces of information on the topic of physical recovery. I found sources that said miscarriage creates minimal physical pain and others that said the symptoms are much more intense. I read that a woman would experience backaches and bleeding and recover quickly, but I also read that it would take several weeks for recovery.

I didn't agree with some sources that implied that a woman didn't need any recovery time nor with others that suggested she couldn't have a successful recovery after a healthy period of time had passed. Often miscarriage mimics real labor, with contractions to expel the fetus. This can be very painful. The truth is that some women will have more intense symptoms of miscarriage than others, hence the confusion. Just as every woman experiences different symptoms in her menstrual cycle and pregnancies, miscarriage symptoms are unique to each woman. Being educated about what you can expect and what you may do to improve your situation will help.

With my first miscarriage, I had no idea what to expect. I hadn't received much instruction from my doctor, and I was sent home with the idea that I would have a heavy period with cramping and that would be it. Unfortunately, I ended up in the emergency room because my cervix was not dilating. I would have liked to have been better prepared. I realize every woman will not have such problems during a miscarriage, but we all need to be aware of the possibilities in order to have the help we desire more readily available.

If you suspect you are going to miscarry, I encourage you to seek advice from your doctor as to the options you have. Ask your doctor what to do if certain situations arise. Most doctors will offer a surgical procedure called dilation and curettage (D&C) to remove the fetal and placental tissue, and they will offer advice and other options on how to handle the miscarriage at home with warnings to contact your physician, or go to the emergency room if there is excessive bleeding or pain.

After a miscarriage, it may be difficult to feel like doing anything. The longer you are inactive, the more you will want to stay that way. After a short period of physical recovery, it is helpful to become involved in activities that are meaningful to you.

If you are in the second or third trimester of pregnancy when miscarriage occurs, you will have to deal with many of the same issues that a normal delivery would entail. Your body may still look pregnant for a few weeks, and your breasts may leak milk. In this case, your doctor will advise you of the types of exercises that are safe. Generally, increasing your activity slowly will help you get back in shape. It is safe to resume sexual activity after the bleeding has stopped.

One of my favorite types of exercise is yoga. It is so adaptable, and there are many levels of difficulty. I enjoy yoga not only because of the physical reward but because of the centering I feel in my body and mind as I practice. I would recommend practicing yoga to get your body back in shape without overdoing it. As you continue to feel better, you can increase the intensity of your exercises. Even going for short walks in the fresh air can help tremendously. Moving is so important. In a sense, you are telling your body to move away from this bad experience toward better health.

A very common misunderstanding about miscarriage in the first trimester is that the miscarriage occurred because of something the mother did physically or something she was exposed to. It is important to dispel these myths because they imply that the woman is at fault for the miscarriage. Only in cases where a person experiences direct trauma to the uterus can miscarriage be linked to physical activity. With few exceptions, pregnant women are encouraged to continue in regular physical activity, even running and other cardiovascular exercise, well into their second trimester.

STAYING ACTIVELY ENGAGED

Heavenly Father has provided one of the greatest remedies for all of our emotional ailments. It is called service to your fellow men. When we are actively engaged in a good cause, it's hard to be consumed with our own personal grief. To serve others is to look outside ourselves and recognize that even though our life may not be in a happy spot, we can still shine a light for others in need.

Everyone on earth suffers at one point or another. Some people seem to suffer more than others, but there are countless stories about those individuals who could be bitter and depressed about their condition but instead are happy and serving others.

Even though our trials may be great, we must remember to look outside ourselves and find the healing balm of service. "And behold, I tell you these things that ye may learn wisdom; that ye may learn that when ye are in the service of your fellow beings ye are only in the service of your God" (Mosiah 2:17). We can pray to have opportunities of service revealed to us. There is always someone in need of a cheerful smile, a kind word, or a good deed. When you are serving others, you will feel the burden of your pain lightened as you seek to be more Christlike.

There have been times in my own life when I have felt my lot was hard, and then I was called upon to serve another person in need. Looking on their situation, whatever it may have been, I decided I would rather endure my own trials than trade with them. One particular situation stands out in my mind.

I was still struggling to find meaning in my childless life and find peace in my trials when I was prompted to serve another. A woman in my ward—I'll call her Carrie—had been sick for quite some time. I had been asked to take a meal to her family even though we had never met. From the outside Carrie did not appear as ill as she was, and I think some people didn't realize the seriousness of her illness.

When I took the meal to her, Carrie answered the door with a smile and greeted me with kindness. We visited for a few minutes, and she thanked me for the meal. A few weeks later, I made a new recipe for dinner that yielded much more than my husband and I could possibly eat. I called another sister in my ward and asked if there might be anyone who could use a meal that day. We both tried to think of someone in need and couldn't think of anyone except Carrie. At first I wondered if I should take another meal to Carrie since it seemed like such a short time since my last visit. Shaking aside my doubt, my husband and I took the meal to Carrie's family and visited with them briefly.

Carrie had several children at home and a son serving a mission. Of course, my husband and I felt the usual joys of service as we returned to our home that evening. The next morning, my friend called and told me Carrie had passed away. My friend commented that the Lord had truly inspired us to serve. I was shocked and could not believe Carrie's family was now without a mother. I thought of the hardships ahead for her family, of the son on the mission who would not get to say good-bye to his mother. I suddenly felt my problems were small in comparison. Overall, I had a feeling of peace that the Lord had allowed me to be a part of Carrie's life so that I could see my own life in a clearer perspective and forget my suffering for a time.

The Lord is willing to help all of us, and we are His best tools to help others. You can create your own miracles of service on a daily basis by being in tune with the Spirit and seeking for opportunities to serve. Continue serving, if possible, in your ward or branch and magnify your callings. You were given a special blessing to fulfill your callings when you were set apart. The Lord knew all you would experience, and He called you to serve despite your trials. Do your visiting and home teaching because when you reach out to others, you are often the beneficiary. Keep active in your family home evenings, family and personal prayer, and scripture study. By living the basic principles of the gospel, you are staying on the path of righteousness and preparing yourself to receive future blessings.

Visit the temple often. One of the most priceless kinds of service we can render is done within the walls of the holy temple. In this time of turmoil in your life, the peace of the temple can soften the blows of your trials. If you are not near a temple, find time to meditate and study about the covenants we make in the temple. Renew your understanding of your baptismal covenants and remember that Heavenly Father wants to help you. Be anxiously engaged in the Lord's work so you will be prepared to have your burdens of sorrow lifted from you.

Getting Pregnant Again

Medically, it is possible for a woman to ovulate and become pregnant within one month after an early miscarriage; however, your doctor may advise you to use contraception for a time to allow your body to recover from the miscarriage.

There are differing opinions on when to try to conceive again. Some doctors recommend that women wait two to three menstrual cycles before trying to get pregnant to give their bodies and psyches time to heal. You need to consult with your doctor as to your individual case and risks. If you are uncertain about your doctor's advice, you may seek out a second opinion.

My first doctor told me to get pregnant again right away, but I didn't feel I was in the proper mental state to do that. My next doctor told me to wait two months. You need to evaluate how you feel. For some it may make sense to try again as soon as possible; for others it may require more time. I think the most important thing you can do is to make this decision as a couple. You may also want to seek the inspiration of the Spirit as you ponder this decision.

Some women have told me they were frightened to try again because of what could happen. Others felt they would be betraying the baby they lost by trying to conceive so soon. These are valid concerns, and I experienced many feelings of confusion as well. Relying on gospel principles and priesthood blessings helped me to sort out my feelings.

Denise shared, "It is okay to mourn, and it is okay to get excited to try to have a baby again. Take a break and get yourself in the best place you can be—physically, mentally, and spiritually—for when you do have another baby. Just reading the scriptures helped me feel better. Every day I would find new inspiration from them." Another woman said, "I think having healthy pregnancies after a miscarriage helps to ease the pain and worry."

I agree that any time we experience success after a failure, we're not as worried that we'll fail again. But some of us will experience other difficulties. Two years after my first miscarriage and after subsequent disappointments month after month, I finally became pregnant again, only to miscarry a second time. After experiencing infertility and a second miscarriage, I was terrified of what could happen. Part of me did not want to try for another pregnancy because I didn't want to experience more pain and loss. I had to look deep inside myself to find the faith to try again. I am forever grateful that my next pregnancy was successful. After nearly five years of marriage, my husband and I were finally able to bring our baby girl home.

I realize there are many couples who are still struggling with infertility and miscarriage. There are some who may not be able to have children during this earth life, but I believe the Lord watches over us and with His omniscient love, He has a plan for each of us.

There are many instances in the scriptures that urge us to rely on faith. In Alma we learn, "Now, as I said concerning faith—that it was not a perfect knowledge—even so it is with my words. Ye cannot know of their surety at first, unto perfection, any more than faith is a perfect knowledge. . . . And now, behold, because ye have tried the experiment, and planted the seed, and it swelleth and sprouteth, and beginneth to grow, ye must needs know that the seed is good. And now, behold, is your knowledge perfect? Yea, your knowledge is perfect in that thing" (32:26, 33–34).

If we have faith and trust that the Lord knows our suffering and yet allows it and still loves us, then perhaps we can remember to rely on Him to provide comfort in our times of need.

When you do become pregnant, do your best to have a healthy pregnancy. Strive to be physically fit and active. Your body will let you know if you are overdoing it, so be ready to listen. Your doctor will advise you if you need to be more careful because of your specific pregnancy. Just because one woman can or cannot do something during her pregnancy does not mean those same guidelines automatically apply to you.

For Malinda, having a miscarriage helped her to pay careful attention to her health and nutrition. "Once I realized I was pregnant again, I also discovered several vitamin and iron deficiencies that might have caused me to miscarry a second time if not for my ever-vigilant doctor. By taking extra vitamins and getting back on a workout routine, I was able to prevent that possibly terrible outcome."

Even our best efforts to be healthy may not guarantee that we will have a successful pregnancy. Unfortunately this may not be in our hands. However, there are some things we can do to help improve our health and reduce the chances for miscarriage. Follow the Word of Wisdom and use sound judgment with everything you eat. You should continue taking folic acid supplements daily if you are considering trying for pregnancy again in the near future. It is also important to avoid caffeine because recent studies have linked caffeine consumption to an increased risk of miscarriage. I encourage you to read the Word of Wisdom, found in Doctrine and Covenants 89, and ponder the counsel the Lord has given us in these last days. Part of that section states,

> And all saints who remember to keep and do these sayings, walking in obedience to the commandments, shall receive health in their navel and marrow to their bones; And shall find wisdom and great treasures of knowledge, even hidden treasures; And shall run and not be weary, and shall walk and not faint. And I, the Lord, give unto them a promise, that the destroying angel shall pass by them, as the children of Israel, and not slay them. Amen. (D&C 89:18–21)

chapter 5

COPING

SPIRITUALLY

THE LORD'S TIMETABLE

Robert C. Oaks said, "We can grow in faith only if we are willing to wait patiently for God's purposes and pattern to unfold in our lives, on His timetable."[1] Heavenly Father is mindful of us. In Doctrine and Covenants 58:2–4, we read about God's designs.

> For verily I say unto you, blessed is he that keepeth my commandments, whether in life or in death; and he that is faithful in tribulation, the reward of the same is greater in the kingdom of heaven. Ye cannot behold with your natural eyes, for the present time, the design of your God concerning those things which shall come hereafter, and the glory which shall follow after much tribulation. For after much tribulation come the blessings. Wherefore the day cometh that ye shall be crowned with much glory; the hour is not yet, but is nigh at hand.

I love the promises contained in those verses, but I have wondered when those blessings will be given. Not all blessings may be realized during our time on earth, but we are promised glory in heaven. It is often difficult to remember that our main purpose on this earth is to prove ourselves worthy of the glory we can receive in heaven.

Following is a quote from a woman who experienced miscarriage. She said, "I learned one very important lesson through this—the Lord sends children when He chooses to. We have a lot less say in the timing than we think we do. It is hard for us to put things in the Lord's hands, but ultimately everything is 'in the Lord's time.'"

Elder Neal A. Maxwell linked patience and faith together when he taught, "Patience is tied very closely to faith in our Heavenly Father. Actually, when we are unduly impatient, we are suggesting that we know what is best—better than does God. Or, at least, we are asserting that our timetable is better than His."[2]

THE REASON WE ARE HERE

Our purpose in coming to earth is to obtain bodies and live our lives such that we can return to be with our Heavenly Father again. We will each have our own trials, and we should strive to overcome them with the faith necessary.

Satan wants us to believe that we didn't choose to come to earth but that God forced us into His plan because He enjoys our suffering. The "father of all lies" wants us to feel that Heavenly Father thinks pain is the only way we can learn. Satan wants us to be angry at the Lord and blame Him for all our troubles and pain. I have to admit that sometimes in the midst of my problems and trials I have jokingly said to my husband, "I'm not sure I signed up for this—I think somebody tricked me." But sadly, many people do believe some distorted view of our Heavenly Father's plan, and their misconceptions keep them from enjoying this life.

I believe we most certainly did understand every facet of our Father's plan in the pre-existence and that we made an educated decision to come to earth. In fact, we fought for it! A plan was created for us to have the opportunity to experience something beyond the premortal world. We were taught about agency and how our right and wrong choices and those of others around us would impact our lives on earth.

Heavenly Father said we would still be His sons and daughters on earth as we were in heaven and that we would have the opportunity to learn who we were and of our individual worth. Our Heavenly Father had confidence that we would make it—that despite the pains and troubles of the earth, we would have the potential to triumph.

Remember in Doctrine and Covenants 122:8 when Joseph Smith is reminded that Christ has gone through the worst of the worst and that He understands our suffering? Like Joseph, we will be supported in our trials if we have the faith necessary. The Lord has the power and will to help us through all of our trials, no matter what they are. Sometimes we choose to turn our backs on the Lord. We give up because we feel the trials are too great, and we let sin and neglect keep us from being close to the Lord. The Lord continues to love us, even if we sometimes forget Him.

Alejandra related: "Heavenly Father loves you and won't let you have any trials greater than you can bear. It helped my hurting to try to be busy doing what I was supposed to and to try to figure out how and what I could learn from the experience."

Just because we have trials doesn't mean we are loved any less. Our Savior is always there, full of unconditional love. We get mad or sad about the necessary trials in our lives, yet we claim to want to be like God. How can we become like Heavenly Father if we have not experienced these things? We need to believe in His plan completely, with no "what ifs" or lack of confidence. If we can make a sincere effort to understand our Father's plan and have faith in His timetable, we will receive a greater understanding of how to endure our trials.

This life and the trials we face might not always seem fair, but God will console the faithful in their trials. It is important to remember that if we are faithful, Jesus Christ will stand with us and plead our cause before Heavenly Father (see D&C 45:3–5).

I found a passage in my journal that I wrote before I had a successful pregnancy.

> I have finally learned to embrace the waiting period the Lord has laid before me and learn from my trials. I have gained strength through the scriptures, particularly Doctrine and Covenants 122:7, "All these things shall give thee experience, and shall be for thy good." This idea is also found in John 16:33, "In the world ye shall have tribulation: but be of good cheer; I have overcome the world." Through many priesthood blessings I have been promised that I will be a mother. I have learned to

accept help from others and find ways to more readily invite the Spirit into my life.

Ecclesiastes 3:1 states, "To every thing there is a season, and a time to every purpose under the heaven." Continue reading in your scriptures through verse 9 to see how specific the Lord is in revealing how many times and seasons there are in our lives.

One of my friends advised me that the best thing I could do was "to pray to be helped through your trials, to understand, to keep perspective, to have faith and hope, and above all to pray that He will bless you in the way that is best for your good."

In the Bible dictionary under the topic of *prayer* we read,

> As soon as we learn the true relationship in which we stand toward God (namely, God is our Father, and we are his children), then at once prayer becomes natural and instinctive on our part. Many of the so-called difficulties about prayer arise from forgetting this relationship. Prayer is the act by which the will of the Father and the will of the child are brought into correspondence with each other. The object of prayer is not to change the will of God, but to secure for ourselves and for others blessings that God is already willing to grant, but that are made conditional on our asking for them.

Many of our prayers may seem to remain unanswered according to the desires of our hearts, but according to the will of the Lord, all prayers are heard. Although the outcomes may not be what we expect, our prayers are answered. In Psalm 145:9 we read, "The Lord is good to all and his tender mercies are over all his works."

Even with all of our understanding, it is very difficult to trust in the Lord's timetable. Communicating with others who have experienced loss can provide insight into your life. In this book, I have included nuggets of wisdom from a number of people. I'm so grateful for Danielle, who shared her experience and offered yet another point of view.

> It's okay to cry and get mad and wonder if you will ever be blessed with the promises that you are entitled to. You are not a bad person for this trial. Heavenly Father is not punishing you for anything you did in the past. Don't look at others, who are able to get pregnant and have babies, with envy. Those babies are not yours. Yours will come one way

or another. There is always a plan, and our plan isn't the way it happens. It is so hard to wait and wonder, but hang in there.

Romans 8:28 reminds us, "And we know that all things work together for good to them that love God, to them who are the called according to his purpose."

I think it's important to find something that draws us closer to our Heavenly Father and that we enjoy. Music is very important to me and to our Father in Heaven. Many kinds of wonderful inspirational music can lift our spirits and give us understanding and strength to endure. Several hymns helped me and continue to lift my spirits each time I listen to them. Even reading the verses provides great insight.

I encourage you to search through the hymn book, read the verses, listen to the music, and find solace for your personal experiences. One hymn that I think relates so much to the questions, suffering, and need for inspiration that those suffering from miscarriage and stillbirth experience is hymn 285, "God Moves in a Mysterious Way." Read through the text and think about your situation. How do the words help you understand your circumstance?

> God moves in a mysterious way
> His wonders to perform;
> He plants his footsteps in the sea
> And rides upon the storm.
>
> Ye fearful Saints, fresh courage take;
> The clouds ye so much dread
> Are big with mercy and shall break
> In blessings on your head.
>
> His purposes will ripen fast,
> Unfolding ev'ry hour;
> The bud may have a bitter taste,
> But sweet will be the flower.
>
> Blind unbelief is sure to err
> And scan his works in vain;
> God is his own interpreter,
> And he will make it plain.[3]

Keeping a journal, writing poetry, and even writing songs helped me move through my grief. I felt more connected with the Spirit when I listened to wholesome music.

As mortals on this earth, we are blessed with fleeting memories. Some of our experiences might be the most painful of our existence, but with time and the Lord's hand, the memory will lose the razor-blade edge of pain. When I was experiencing my struggle to have children, I felt I would never get over some of the things that happened to me. It seemed my heart was rebreaking every other day, and even though I tried to remain strong, I wasn't strong enough. But I realize now that as I kept striving to live righteously and keep my covenants, the unhappy memories began to fade.

When I became pregnant for the second time, I was ecstatic, but the excitement was short-lived. I began spotting only seven weeks into the pregnancy. I remember that we hadn't told anyone I was pregnant, and I wasn't planning to tell until I was sure things were okay. I dreaded having to give people the news that I was going to miscarry again.

Over the weekend, we traveled home for my brother's missionary homecoming, and we were not going to tell anyone I was pregnant. But because of complications, we decided to tell them. It was awful for me to tell my family that I was pregnant, but that I would probably lose this baby as well. I asked for a special blessing from my husband, dad, brother, and brother-in-law. After the blessing, I knew that I would miscarry. I was so discouraged that we actually drove back home right after church so that we would miss the large celebration with friends and family. I just couldn't bear to answer one more time, the question, "So, when are you going to have kids?"

After I returned home, I went to the doctor. He ran some tests and did an ultrasound that confirmed I would miscarry again. We scheduled a D&C procedure (dilation and curettage) to avoid the complications I experienced with my first miscarriage. Other than being emotionally crushed, I physically felt well enough to continue working until my scheduled hospital visit. In all honesty, I didn't have much of a choice because I owned a cleaning business that was in charge of cleaning over eighty apartments within a ten-day period. So I went to work to finish up the job.

While I was working, one of my friends asked me about our family planning. She knew about my earlier miscarriage, and I told her that I was currently having another miscarriage. She was shocked by my answer, but managed to say she was sorry.

At the same time, one of my nieces had just been diagnosed with possible cancer in her leg. I remember praying to Heavenly Father and pleading with all my might that she would be all right. My life was an emotional roller coaster at that point.

It was the Tuesday after Mother's Day when we finished cleaning the apartments. As I left the apartment building, the owners asked me if I'd had a happy Mother's Day and then asked if I had any children. It's hard to describe how painful it was to answer politely, "No," while thinking to myself that in two days I would go to the hospital to have my second pregnancy failure taken care of.

If someone had told me then that the memory of this painful episode would fade with time and not hurt so fiercely, I'm not sure I would have believed them. But it is true. The memory doesn't hurt now, and though I can read my detailed journal account of my feelings at that time and remember, I realize that I now have a different perspective.

Everything went well with my procedure, and my niece experienced a miracle when, after much fasting and prayer, another examination found no cancer in her leg. At the time all of this was going on, my father-in-law said that the Lord must have something pretty good in store for us because we kept getting all kinds of trials.

I realize why we have been commanded to keep a personal record of our lives. It was so helpful during this time to go back and read about how I felt and how I handled my first miscarriage. At the time of my second miscarriage, I wrote the following:

> I have been reading from my past journal about my first miscarriage. Steve and I really went through some terrible times. I was very depressed and unhappy. I had lost my direction in life. I feel like I'm doing a lot better this time. I just feel a peacefulness that is hard to explain. I know I never thought I could survive another tragedy like the first miscarriage, but I know my Savior is carrying me through this one. Steve and I have grown so much. We get along so much better now. Steve is the best husband, and I think we are both dealing with this miscarriage better.

I have a hope that we will have a baby soon. It is very painful, but I am trying to be patient. I look back at how very awful I felt after my first miscarriage, and I feel like a different person now. I feel stronger and am so grateful for the power of the priesthood. The blessing I received with anointing oil really prepared me for this trial. Sometimes it's hard to see our blessings through all the trials. But we do have many blessings. You just can't compare yourself to other people because their lives always look so easy in comparison. But we would probably not want their trials either. I know that life will get better!

Mine is a success story, but not just because I have children now. It is because I came through my trials with my testimony of the gospel still intact and even stronger than it was before. It was a hard road, a long road, and there were many painful detours, but I have finally arrived at a place where the knowledge of my Savior's love for me will help me to continue through the journey of my life.

My trials are not over now because I have children. Many would say they are just beginning! Understanding that the Lord has a plan for each of us and that He willingly provides us with so many tools to travel through life successfully is what makes all the difference.

Notes
1. Robert C. Oaks, "The Power of Patience," *Ensign*, Nov. 2006, 16–17.
2. Neal A. Maxwell, "Patience," *Ensign*, Oct. 1980, 28.
3. *Hymns*, "God Moves in a Mysterious Way," 285.

chapter 6

No Child to Hold

Coping with Miscarriage and Infertility

After I experienced my first miscarriage, I heard all kinds of horror stories about people who had experienced several miscarriages in a row. My worst fear was that I would miscarry again. But then I realized an even greater fear—that I might not be able to get pregnant again.

Month after month went by, and I held onto the hope that this time I would be pregnant. I took several pregnancy tests when I was only one day late because I wanted so fervently to see that positive sign.

Every time a new cycle started, signaling another failure, the disappointment was overwhelming. I was consumed with trying to get pregnant and was so hyper-aware of any anticipated symptoms. Looking back, I think I was a crazy lady to actually want to be nauseous. Thankfully, I can smile about it now even though I still wish I would have felt happier then. I was a pretty good cover artist. I tried not to let people see how much I was hurting or what I was suffering from. I felt as if I was continually deflecting all kinds of hurtful comments on a regular basis.

"So when are you guys gonna have kids?" someone would ask, and I would cringe inwardly but smile and say, "We're working on it." I felt so exposed when asked that question, and I had to think up an appropriate response because I didn't want to say, "Well, I had a miscarriage and now I can't get pregnant. Thanks for asking. How's your life going?"

I started to fall into that rut I've since heard about from so many women—a deep fissure of disappointment, resentment, bitterness, and sadness. Everywhere around me were happy little families with cute children. I also saw many instances of unwanted or neglected children and wondered why the Lord would not bless me with a baby. I had forgotten about the promises of our Heavenly Father's plan.

My husband and I started discussing adoption. We had no idea how we would ever be able to afford it and again felt discouraged as our dreams of having children seemed to be further away each month. We both grieved in different ways, and I retreated further into a protective shell I had built around me as my means of survival.

It was hard to talk to each other because the only thing we were really interested in was having a baby, and it was depressing to focus on our infertility. At the same time, we needed to talk to each other because we were the only ones, it seemed, who understood what was happening in our lives. No one in my family had experienced a miscarriage, and although they were very supportive, they couldn't help me understand my situation. I felt lost and had so many questions. It seemed every other day someone was asking me about the most private part of my life and expecting me to tell all.

During this time, I learned a very important lesson. One of my close friends had gone through an extended period of infertility with surgeries, treatments, and medications to try to conceive. I remembered how I had once asked her some of the same insensitive questions people were now asking me. I felt awful as I realized that I had inflicted pain on her when she was already suffering. I realized that sometimes people just don't know what to say. We're not all gifted conversationalists, and our mouths often run faster than they should. I recognized that I had likely hurt my friend's feelings, just as my own feelings had been injured. It was an important moment for me because I realized I was actually learning something from my trials.

Linda experienced infertility and shared her story.

It took us nine years before we finally started our family. I would have liked it to be one year. I couldn't understand why this had happened to me. Why was I being punished? And worse, why was my husband being punished because I wasn't able to give him children? That probably felt the worst—that I couldn't give him something he so badly wanted. I also know he felt the same way toward me, since the doctor never could tell us why we couldn't conceive.

After years and years of trying, we went to a specialist and did everything we could except in vitro fertilization, and that was only because it would have cost over ten grand and it wasn't guaranteed. I had reached the point where I was tired of trying—physically and emotionally drained. Then I came across a friend who told me about her adoption experience, and the doors opened for me! A year or so later my husband came around to the idea, and we knew this was how we were to have our family. What an experience adoption was!

Linda also shared with me how her life was blessed in a completely unexpected way.

We love our two little girls who are eight days apart and who came to us from two different birth mothers, and we love those women who brought them into the world and entrusted us to be the parents to their beautiful babies. Adoption is an amazing option for those who feel as we did, and I hope others will look at adoption earlier than we did. I know we love them as though they were our own, but I guarantee that we love them more because we travelled down such a long and hard road to finally get our precious babies. We won't ever take our family for granted, and for that I am truly grateful for this trial.

Coping with infertility is very difficult. One thing I would tell myself if I could go back in time is to be happy and keep living my life to the fullest extent possible. Instead of being mired down in disappointment, I wish I could've told myself to fully take advantage of my waiting period to improve myself physically, emotionally, and spiritually. There were many times when I thought about getting involved in something that would have been good for me, but then I thought, *Well, I might be pregnant before I finish this class or project or whatever, so I better not do it.*

Keep growing!

I wish I could go back and tell myself to focus on all my blessings and opportunities instead of the lack of them. I'm sure if I could go back, it would be very hard to convince my past self that I was blessed at all. It would be like putting a shiny new bike in front of a child and telling him to think about a skateboard instead. Or maybe pulling a brand-new sports car into the garage and telling someone not to drive it but to take up running.

When we are focused solely on something we want but can't have, even if it is a righteous desire, we may miss other blessings Heavenly Father is willing to give us. It's important to keep a broader perspective of life and its many seasons. If we can try to remember that there are specific blessings in store for us, we will experience more happiness during our waiting period.

Felicia gave me a wonderful example of this. "Having to face the fact that I may never have any more children has been devastating. I have come to the point in this trial that I have had to turn it all over to the Lord. I have let Him know that I want more kids and that I am not okay with only two. But I have told Him that if I am only meant to have two kids, then to please help me to be all right with that. Since I have done this, the pain is not as bad, and I feel a bit better."

It is very difficult to understand the Lord's timetable and why events unfold as they do. After dealing with the frustrating experience of infertility, it seemed I would never understand my trials. I have since learned of an experience I think is enlightening.

Nathan was turning nineteen and was worthy to serve a mission. He excitedly filled out his papers and anxiously awaited his mission call. He had been a member his entire life and had prepared for this time of service. After a period of time, Nathan received a letter from the First Presidency of the Church, but it was a very different letter than the one he expected. This letter informed Nathan that although he was worthy and prepared to go on a mission, the Lord did not see fit to call him at this time. He was told that he must wait and remain faithful to the Lord.

Imagine how difficult it must have been for Nathan to return to his church-owned university and attend classes with other students who curiously looked his way as he approached his twentieth birthday and did not go on a mission. Many girls would not date him because they assumed he was unworthy to serve a mission. When Nathan did meet a girl who wanted to get to know him, her parents were strongly against their daughter dating a young man who had not served a mission. At this time, Nathan decided to show his letter to the family to prove he was indeed worthy to serve a mission but that the Lord had other plans for him which had not yet been revealed. It was a great trial for Nathan to walk down a different path than he had expected, but he kept his faith and continued to serve the Lord and live righteously. He was recently married in the temple to his beautiful bride.

Nathan still doesn't understand exactly why he was not called to serve a mission, but as he was counseled—he remained faithful to the Lord. Nathan had a letter to prove why his circumstance was different from others. I was promised in numerous blessings that I would be a mother, and my patriarchal blessing also mentioned motherhood, but I didn't know when or how that would happen. While I struggled with miscarriage and infertility, there were many times I wished I had a letter that proved my worthiness to be a mother. I often doubted my individual worth and wondered if I was strong enough to make it through my trials. Sometimes I wished I could wear a sign for others' benefit that said, "No, I'm not pregnant and I don't know when we're going to be able to start our family—it is in the Lord's hands, and it will happen in His time."

Now I realize I did not need a letter. All I needed was to have strong enough faith to withstand my trials and not doubt that my Heavenly Father would fulfill the promises He had made to me. Although I had to walk a different path than the one I had planned for or the one that I felt was most desirable, it did not mean the Lord loved me any less. As long as we can hold to the iron rod, no matter what different obstacles we may encounter, we will still end up where our Heavenly Father wants us to be.

Julie B. Beck said: "In my experience I have seen that some of the truest mother hearts beat in the breasts of women who will not rear their own children in this life, but they know that 'all things must come to pass in their time' and that they 'are laying the foundation of a great work' (D&C 64:32–33)."[1]

Notes:
1. Julie B. Beck, "A 'Mother Heart,'" *Ensign*, May 2004, 76.

chapter 7

Experiencing Miscarriage and Infertility after the Birth of a Child

Even though many people have experienced miscarriages, the circumstances of a miscarriage are different for each couple and each time it happens. For example, it is a different situation when you miscarry or experience infertility after the birth of a child. I think just knowing that someone recognizes your specific loss is a very helpful step in your recovery.

We have already covered the lack of understanding or sympathy that sometimes accompanies miscarriage. I have noticed that this problem seems to increase if you have a child and then experience problems. I have heard time and time again that people would comment, "At least you have one," like that was supposed to offer comfort.

The most common response I gathered from others was that people think you shouldn't mourn because you already have a baby. A question I would like to pose for anyone who doesn't understand this concept is, if you had two children and I took one of them away, do you think you shouldn't miss him because you already have one child?

If you have a child or children and then experience a miscarriage or infertility, it is still a loss. Many women have experienced this unfortunate event. Here is Teresa's story.

> I married at age twenty and got pregnant two and a half years later, after a few months of trying. Other than horrible morning sickness and being huge at the end, I had a perfect pregnancy. Infertility never crossed my mind. A few years later, we decided to try for another child, and I had a positive pregnancy test. Two weeks later, I lost the baby. We continued to try for a baby and over the course of the next year, I experienced two more miscarriages. My husband and I agreed to try one more time. On July 24th, one day late, just like her sister, she joined us and is now a feisty twenty-month-old, who loves to go outside. My girls are three weeks shy of being four years apart.

Even after having three successful pregnancies, I know nothing is guaranteed. When I think about having more children, I hope I will have enough faith to know that the Lord's hand is in all things. I am still not sure of myself and because I live among many Latter-day Saints, by the time my first child was fifteen months, I was already being asked when we were going to have more children. This was stressful for me because I was worried about the future too. I didn't really need an extra reminder from someone else. Every time someone asked, I tried not to focus on the problems I had experienced in the past. It was difficult because I knew that everything doesn't always go like clockwork.

Creating your family is one of the most personal and sacred events of your life. Unfortunately, some people feel it is their business to know the full extent of your family planning. I hope that anyone who reads this book will understand this is a private matter. If you are well acquainted with the person and you are both comfortable talking about having kids, then I think it's fine to engage in this type of conversation, but please be respectful of others' privacy.

For example, I was talking with two women and as a conversation usually does, it turned toward children. One woman commented that she had six children and then asked how many we had. I told her I had two, and the other woman said she had one.

"You only have one?" the first woman asked.

We were mere acquaintances, but in a split-second I knew this other woman was struggling. I could see on her face the anguish as she answered, "Yes." I deflected the question and its hurtful assumptions by laughing and telling the lady with six kids, "We're in awe of you. Some of us have to work a little harder to get those children here. It took me a while to get my kids."

Immediately, the tension dissolved, and I could almost feel the woman sitting next to me breathe again. Then she asked me about my children and volunteered that she was experiencing infertility. Only at that time did I ask her anything about her situation. If we can try a little harder to pay close attention to the people we interact with, we will be able to discern how we can lighten their load instead of adding to it.

It's also a good idea not to assume that just because a woman has children, she will automatically know how to deal with a miscarriage. I found that women who had children and experienced miscarriage had many of the same questions as women without children. Noreen said, "I wish I had known more about what was happening to my body. I'd given birth twice before this, and my miscarriage was very different from the labors I'd experienced. I had a great deal of pain but didn't actually start spotting until several days later. When I rushed to the doctor, it was already too late."

No matter what the circumstance may be, miscarriage is still a loss. If you have no children, two children, or ten children, you have still experienced a loss. Refer to Chapter 3 for more information on this subject.

HELPING CHILDREN DEAL WITH A MISCARRIAGE

How do you help your children understand something you can barely comprehend? When you have children and then experience a miscarriage, it is often difficult to explain. A young child can begin to grasp that there is a baby in mommy's tummy, but it takes much more comprehension for them to understand why that baby is suddenly gone.

It's important to acknowledge that even a very young child will recognize a change in his parents' emotions. Children can recognize emotions when they are less than a year old. Your child will notice that Mommy is sad and wonder why.

I have noticed that my children are like little extensions of myself with sensory tools that can quickly adapt to any situation. When I am happy, it is easy for them to be happy. When I am sad or frustrated, their moods reflect mine. I remember a story a woman shared about this very subject. She said one day she felt tired and frustrated, and she snapped at her husband. Then their teenage son came in, sensed the tension, and smacked his little brother. The little boy grew angry and walked over and kicked the cat. This example is a good reminder of how our children are affected by the mood in the home.

In the event of a miscarriage, you and your family may experience a wide variety of emotions. It's important to help your children understand that they are not the cause of your sadness. Remind yourself of how attuned they are to their surroundings, and pray for help to be extra sensitive with them during this time. Heavenly Father can inspire you with wonderful ways to help your family through this trial. Be truthful with your children but adjust your explanations for their ages and comprehension levels.

Brianne experienced four miscarriages and shared how she and her husband relied on the Spirit each time to decide how to help their children through the situation. They felt their children were too young to understand when they experienced their first miscarriage, but, she said, "With the second one, we told them. We both felt very strongly that we needed to. We just explained to them that I had a baby in my tummy, but it was not there anymore. The third time we did not tell them. We only said my tummy was sick. We did not feel we should tell them. I don't know why we felt the way we did, but I think you need to listen to the Spirit to know what to do."

Although the situation may not seem ideal, you can find many great teaching tools from your trials. Brenda shared her experience.

> Right now my kids want a baby. We have talked with them about praying for a baby. Every night they both ask for a baby in their individual prayers as well as in family prayers. One day my son asked why

we couldn't have a baby. Why didn't Heavenly Father want us to have a baby? We then had to discuss trials and how they make us stronger and how we will love a baby so much more. This also brought faith into the discussion. Now that we have been praying for a baby, we have added to bless us with faith to have a baby. My kids are still little enough to not understand, but I am so grateful for the opportunity to be able to have this faith discussion and to grow together as a family.

Having special family home evenings to explain the plan of salvation, faith, the test of our mortal life, and other topics can also help to sustain the testimony of the family. This trial can be a wonderful opportunity to teach children about the attributes of Christ. We can teach about compassion and sympathy and how to help those who are hurting or sad. Having discussions tailored to the age of your children will help with the confusion that may surround the miscarriage.

Staying close to the Lord as we live the gospel to the best of our ability will help our children to cope with stressful events in life. I think it's okay to let your children see your sadness. You don't need to pretend that life is perfect all the time. When children see that it is normal for you to express emotions, it helps them in turn to deal with and express their own feelings.

chapter 8

FOR THOSE WHO COMFORT

How do we comfort someone who has experienced a miscarriage or stillbirth? What can we do to help them? How can we show our love and concern?

In John 11, we read about a miracle Jesus Christ performed. He raised Lazarus from the dead. But before He did this, He mourned with those who mourned in a simple yet beautiful way. In verses 32–35 we read, "Then when Mary was come where Jesus was, and saw him, she fell down at his feet, saying unto him, Lord, if thou hadst been here, my brother had not died. When Jesus therefore saw her weeping, and the Jews also weeping which came with her, he groaned in the spirit, and was troubled, And said, Where have ye laid him? They said unto him, Lord, come and see. Jesus wept."

Jesus did not give Mary explanations or perfect answers at that time; He merely wept with her. He wept with those who were suffering from the pains of losing their loved one. Even though Christ knew what would come, He still wept with them. He did not tell them, "Do not cry for all will be well." Christ offered another miracle at this time as He taught us how to mourn with those that mourn.

As I gathered questions, thoughts, and stories of people's trials for this book, I learned many things. One of the most important is that we are all different. Yes, we already know that, but the fact that we're different means that we all cope with things differently. We all face our grief and trials differently. What comforts one might offend another. That seems confusing, and you may say, "Then how will I ever know what to do?"

The best advice I can think of is to kneel down and ask Heavenly Father how you can help the person in need. The Lord wants to help the people you are comforting, and you are His proxy to serve others. Consider the suggestions given here and pray to know what would work best for the people you know. Remember that grief has many stages. Sometimes people may be at a point where nothing seems to help. However, you can still pray for them. Be aware that they are hurting and that even though they may not accept what you do for them now, this does not mean they won't remember it later. Pray to be able to understand each person (including her personality and characteristics) so you will better be able to help and give her needed support.

The overwhelming response I received from others was that it is easier to talk to someone who had been through the same specific trial. Women who had suffered a miscarriage felt more comfortable talking to those who had also suffered a miscarriage. This makes sense in terms of the Lord's plan and gives us a greater understanding of why we go through trials. It is not only for our personal growth, but so that we may be of greater help to others who have the same type of experiences. A person who has lived through a similar ordeal can empathize at a deeper level, though someone who has not suffered the same type of trial may still offer sincere, heartfelt sympathy.

I don't want you to feel like you can't offer comfort to another just because you haven't suffered through the same ordeal. I think it helps to recognize the difference between empathy and sympathy because when you do, you can better understand why so many women said they appreciated talking to someone who had experienced a miscarriage.

The most important thing you should remember is to care—but be cautious. This topic of bringing children into the world is very private and personal. Some people may not mind sharing their plans for having children, but resist the urge to be a meddler and bite back those nosy questions. After my experience with miscarriages and infertility, I became aware of how often a well-meaning person asked these personal questions. Those who should be most attentive and sensitive to our needs sometimes forget this in their curiosity. Many women feel they can barely get their youngest to the age of two before the questioning begins on when they are going to add another child to the family.

I have been surprised many times by how many people have asked me, "When are you going to have another one?" I often respond, "I don't know." Because I don't, and it scares me to think about the possibilities, given my history. My own desire for a family puts more than enough pressure on me without the additional pressure from curious questioners.

What Should I Say?

Being a good listener and giving a simple acknowledgement are often the best ways to comfort someone you don't know well. But what if it's your best friend, sister, or daughter? You may need to say more when she calls to talk to you. If this happens, you might try saying, "I'm here for you, whenever you want to talk." "That must be so hard." "I'm sure you're really hurting right now." "I'm sorry." Or, "I will pray for you."

I especially liked what my friend Jen said: "I don't know how you feel, but I know how it feels to love a baby." Another woman said, "I don't have words to take away your sorrow, but I'm here for you."

The most important comfort you can give is to acknowledge that they are suffering and that the miscarriage happened. Don't just avoid the subject or them completely. Tiffany shared how she felt about the lack of comfort she experienced. "For me, there was almost no one—including my husband—who seemed to understand that I had lost something very valuable. I tried to make people care, but it was just too exhausting. I really mostly felt alone during that time—and angry because everyone I loved blew it off as 'not meant to be.' I wanted that baby, and they didn't understand why I hurt so badly."

Following are some examples of what helped others.

> A simple "I'm sorry" card or small flower arrangement really helped me. It was more to know people cared than anything else. It seems like the world has ended to a mother who has lost a child, but many people don't understand how you could have bonded with "a few cells." A mother's love begins the day the pregnancy test comes back positive. When I called to talk to people, I didn't really expect them to say much. "How are you?" "How are you feeling today?" "I'm so sorry." And then just listen.

Celia said, "I loved when other ward members came out of the woodwork to comfort me—telling me of their miscarriages. I had no idea how common it was, but felt very loved and understood; they were so sensitive to me because they had been through it."

Most people said they didn't really want to talk at length to someone who hadn't experienced a miscarriage, but you can be a listening ear or a sounding board and just be there for them if they need you. For many, talking to someone who had gone through the same thing and then gone on to have more children seemed to be particularly helpful.

I hope everyone will remember that there is always an opportunity to offer comfort, support, and sympathy. One of the things that hurt the most after my first miscarriage was when I would see people, particularly family members, who knew all about it but didn't say anything or pretended like nothing had happened.

In comparison, it would be like seeing someone with a cast on his arm and never asking, "Are you okay?" Now I realize that they didn't know what to say and were afraid of saying the wrong thing. But because they were a part of my family, I knew that they knew all about my miscarriage and hospital care, so I felt ignored when they said nothing. On the other hand, I didn't want too many prying questions, and I was scared of what they might say. When offering comfort, you have to walk such a fine line, but I still think it's best to acknowledge that the person is suffering, even if it's awkward or painful.

I think if we ask our Heavenly Father for help and then say something comforting to the person suffering, we will have helped in some way. We never know how much little acts of caring and kindness may affect someone. We don't have to talk to them for hours or even minutes. We can just acknowledge that they are suffering. I remember I was touched when one of my extended family members asked, "How are you doing?" I knew what he meant, and I knew it was his way of expressing his love and sympathy for my situation.

I think everyone goes through the grieving process in a different way. Our most intense trials are like a refiner's fire. Some of us more easily rise above offensive comments and uncomfortable situations, while others stop in their progression and are unable to cope with their circumstances. It helps to recognize and be aware of what we shouldn't say as well as what we could or should say.

Try to avoid saying, "I know exactly how you feel." Even if you have been through a similar situation, everyone feels things differently. Be willing to listen to their grief and then, if prompted, offer how you felt in a similar situation.

Again, don't be nosy and don't ask, "So when are you going to have another baby?" One person who responded to my surveys said she felt she had to have her friends tell people in the ward that she had experienced a miscarriage because, she said, "an LDS family with an almost-two-year-old is open to ward speculation." Having children is a commandment of the Lord, but the appropriate number and timing of children in each family is determined by the husband and wife and the Lord.

Don't diminish another person's suffering. Instead, acknowledge that she may be experiencing feelings she doesn't even understand. If someone has suffered a pregnancy loss, please don't ever say, "It's better this way; it probably would have had birth defects." That line of reasoning doesn't offer any comfort.

Remember that this person is hurting, and even though she may try hard to be strong, her feelings are probably still very tender. Think of how Christ would act toward us in our suffering, and how He would probably want to take us in His arms and comfort us. He would know of the terrible pain we felt in our hearts and do all He could to help succor us in our time of need.

WHAT SHOULD I DO?

When your loved one suffers from a miscarriage, it is difficult to know what to say. Sometimes the small acts of service we provide speak louder than words. Marsha related this experience:

> One of the things I appreciated most were the people who just did something instead of asking what I needed. (My answer was always, "Nothing, we're fine.") My Relief Society president came and took my car to vacuum it out and wash it. Another friend weeded my flower bed while another gave us a gift card for Pizza Hut so I could have a night without making dinner. These were things which weren't essential and didn't *have* to be done, but made me feel loved because I knew they cared. The people who hurt me were the ones who didn't know what to say, so they avoided me for a while.

Tanya said, "One friend who had a surprise pregnancy came to me before she told anyone else. She apologized to me. She said 'It's not fair.' She didn't have to do this, but it was the best thing she could have done for me." This is not to imply that everyone has to come to you first to get permission to be pregnant. It just displays how a thoughtful friend considered how she would have felt in that situation. It was probably much easier for Tanya to hear it from her friend personally than in a big gathering where Tanya would have had to display a positive reaction.

Here are a few more examples of acts of service that helped those who were suffering.

+ One thing I did when my sister had a miscarriage was to mark the due date on my calendar and send her flowers that day. I know that was a day she dreaded, and by then most people had forgotten about it and she felt like no one else remembered.
+ Another thing that has really touched me are the few people who have remembered the date and emailed me or called to tell me they are thinking of us.
+ A good friend or sister can also suggest getting out together.

Having a friend to go places with made it easier to face the world again. Offer a ride to enrichment, a walk in the park, or just go together to a store that is having a good sale that week. A burden shared is a burden halved.

- I found much comfort in the priesthood blessings I received. Husbands may offer to give blessings and continue to willingly give as many as are necessary. The Lord does not have an allotted number of priesthood blessings we can receive.

- The one bright spot I remember was the day one of my girlfriends stopped by and brought me lunch. She didn't need to say anything—she was pregnant too and already showing— she just sat with me while I cried.

There is no happy pill or quick fix, but time can heal our wounds. Don't try to rush someone through their grieving process. Just like a broken bone needs weeks to mend, people suffering from a miscarriage will need time to heal. You should allow them the time they need. You can, however, continue to be a source of encouragement and help.

You may become aware of your loved one falling into depression. If within a few weeks she still isn't getting up and getting dressed in the morning, or if she can't face even the simplest tasks, she may need to seek evaluation and help for depression.

Clinical depression is usually defined as prolonged symptoms of depression that may have been triggered by a highly stressful situation or other major life event. It is normal to exhibit some early warning signs of depression. People who suffer a miscarriage experience a major stress in their lives. If, however, they cannot recover from their experience within a reasonable amount of time, then professional help may be needed.

Another aspect to consider is the person who has experienced miscarriage and is now pregnant again. I think it's important to share excitement with them about their new pregnancy. Everyone was so worried when I got pregnant for the third time after experiencing two miscarriages. I remember people asking, "Will you be able to keep this one?"

It hurt to hear this because I had received a blessing in which I was told I would have a healthy pregnancy and be able to have this baby. I had faith that everything would be okay. I wished everyone could be excited with me. I understood they were worried, but I wished they could forget about it for a moment and just have hope for the future.

Each of us has dealt with some form of loss, even if it's not miscarriage. Think of times when you have experienced loss and how you felt. Pondering on those experiences may help you to comfort your loved one with added empathy. We have many examples in the scriptures of the Savior providing comfort to those who were suffering. He commanded us to mourn with those that mourn. As we strive to emulate this Christlike attribute and seek guidance from the Spirit, we will be able to provide help and comfort to others.

chapter 9

Husbands Have a Right to Grieve

Whenever someone mentions miscarriage, our thoughts usually turn to the woman who is suffering. She has gone through a terrible experience, and we try our best to help and comfort her. But what about her husband?

Husbands also have the right and need to mourn. They may experience some of the same or different emotions as their spouses. From my own experience, I remember I was so overwhelmed by my initial grief and pain that I couldn't focus on anything else. I am so grateful that my husband was able to explain to me that he was hurting too. Because he was willing to confide in me, my perspective shifted significantly so I was able to see that the suffering was not just my own, but ours to endure together. It helped me to know that not only was my husband concerned about me, but he too was grieving the loss of our baby.

My husband was not always as verbal about his feelings as I was. There were days when I would forget he was grieving because he mourned in such a quiet way. Men are very different from women emotionally, and particularly in how those emotions are expressed. Women usually find it therapeutic to verbalize their thoughts and emotions, whereas men tend to resolve them by thinking them out and bringing them to a mental resolution. Our differences can and should complement each other, instead of causing discord.

Many women shared with me that their husbands wished someone would acknowledge that they were hurting too. During my research, I have learned that many husbands often felt overlooked and forgotten during the mourning and comforting process. One man said, "It was my baby too and I am hurting just as much as my wife. I know it's different, but I'm not only hurting for the loss of the baby. I'm hurting for the pain my wife is going through."

Even though husbands do have a need and a right to grieve, most will grieve differently than their wives. Because a woman experiences all of the physical changes of pregnancy and miscarriage, it is often hard for her husband to identify with the same emotions. He will likely feel grief, but he may not express his feelings as openly. I talked to many husbands who felt they needed to be strong for their wives and family. Some felt that if they could temper their hurt and disappointment, it would help their wives deal with the situation better.

Unfortunately, this approach may create tension in a marriage at a critical time. Don't hesitate to speak to your husband about his feelings. Give him permission to share his grief. Let him know that the greatest support he can give is in sharing his feelings and identifying with your family's loss. I spoke with a woman who shared some of the difficulties she and her husband faced. She said,

> I wish I would've been more able to help my husband cope. He covered it up and spent all his energy taking care of my physical and emotional needs. He even said, "Maybe you weren't pregnant at all. Maybe the tests were wrong." This just made me angry! I realized later that this was just his way of dealing with it at the time. However, much later, when I believe he finally came to terms with his feelings, he became depressed and made bad choices I don't think he would have made had he dealt with the miscarriage when it happened. I wish I had been more aware of how to help him cope.

One husband said that after his wife's miscarriage, it was hard for him because it affected him differently. She was very sad and was coping as best she could. He didn't want to be insensitive, but he found a different way of coping with the situation by relying on his testimony of the Lord's plan. He said, "It didn't affect me as much. I've always had a strong belief that the Lord knows best and is in control of these types of situations. I do not believe they are random, or accidents. I really believe there is a purpose behind them. I just wish I knew what that purpose was, other than the one of having to go through trials."

Sonya shared some of the feelings she and her husband had as they coped with multiple miscarriages.

> My husband felt each miscarriage was a fluke, and it was difficult to get him to believe that trying over and over again wouldn't fix it. This caused stress in our marriage. He did not mourn as much as I did and was ready to announce the last pregnancy much earlier than I was. I can't imagine trying to support someone so close to you when they are going through this. He couldn't really do anything, but he was always there. For my two horrible first trimesters, he cooked every meal.

Amanda said,

> Since we already had two children, my husband kind of shrugged it off and said, "Well, guess we weren't meant to have that one." He wasn't trying to be insensitive, but he didn't know what to say to me. He didn't seem to realize—I doubt he does even now—that my heart ached with loss as strong as if someone had died. I cried alone, I grieved alone, and I suffered alone. I needed my husband's love and his strong arms of comfort, and because he truly didn't understand, he wasn't able to offer those things.

Even in the face of these differences, we can cleave to one another and help each other through our trials. Marriage is such a beautiful part of the plan of salvation because we can help each other through every experience. Rather than standing alone, trying to fight feelings of despair, we can turn to each other and walk together through the pains of this earth. In the scriptures we read, "Therefore shall a man leave his father and his mother, and shall cleave unto his wife: and they shall be one flesh" (Genesis 2:24). If you use this opportunity to become closer, your marriage will be stronger, and you will be better prepared for the trials you may face in the future.

Elaine shared how miscarriage affected her husband. "He was devastated by it as well. I did not realize just how much he was affected until a bit later. We really had to lean on each other. Nobody else understood what we were going through. We would hold hands more and sit by each other more often. It brought us so much closer."

It may be helpful for couples to seek assistance from their doctor, a counselor, their bishop, family, and friends and also to pray to Heavenly Father together to seek His comfort and guidance. It may be difficult for spouses to communicate their emotional needs to one another, but that doesn't mean the needs are not there. With time and patience, you can work through this trial together. Stay close to the Lord and strive to be unselfish and patient as you work out your individual and collective feelings. Seek comfort from the ultimate Comforter. Pray together, read the scriptures together, attend the temple together, and continue to fulfill your Church callings and be faithful members of the Church.

Our marriages may seem to take a beating when we go through trials because of the different ways men and women cope with situations. Unfortunately many couples develop significant marital problems in conjunction with infertility and child-bearing difficulties. The very thing they were striving so hard for ends up ultimately driving them apart. Remembering that Heavenly Father is an integral part of our sacred union can help us realize how powerful the marriage bond is.

I encourage you to look outside your current situation and see that your marriage will continue well beyond your present problems. If you have a firm foundation, you will be able to endure your trials. Finding ways to serve each other and make life a little easier for each other will keep the love of your marriage alive.

Looking back at my situation, I know I could have handled some things differently. It would have helped me if I had realized that no matter what my husband's reactions were to our situation, he did love me dearly. I wish I had remembered that just because I was in physical and emotional pain and was very vocal about it, did not mean my husband wasn't suffering alongside me in his quiet way.

Through those early years of disappointment and grief, my husband was always there for me. He didn't always know just how to help, but he was always available to hold me and help me through my tears. I'm so grateful my husband saw the potential in our marriage and held on tight to the promises we had made, even in the face of difficulty. I am also grateful I did not choose to withdraw from him emotionally or physically during those difficult times. Keeping the lines of communication open and not being afraid to share our feelings has supported our marriage through this and many other trials.

chapter 10

We are all of Infinite Worth

"And God saw these souls that they were good, and he stood in the midst of them, and he said: These I will make my rulers; for he stood among those that were spirits, and he saw that they were good; and he said unto me: Abraham, thou art one of them; thou wast chosen before thou wast born" (Abraham 3:23).

As Latter-day Saints, when we think about death in general, we are comforted by the knowledge of the plan of salvation and our testimony of the hereafter. Even though we know that if we are righteous we will be with our deceased loved ones again, it is still difficult.

Some people may be able to cope better than others, based on their stage in life. The way we mourn often reflects our level of knowledge and understanding of gospel truths and how they affect us individually. Although we have not been given the same exact reassurances with miscarriage as we have been with the death of a loved one, the plan of salvation still offers comfort and hope. And we will eventually come to know that there is a purpose for what we have experienced.

Heavenly Father loves us unconditionally, especially in the face of our trials. He knows our individual worth and our potential. For some reason, when we are faced with seemingly unending trials, we may feel that our Father doesn't love us. He does, and He knows exactly how we will benefit from our trials. He is the master sculptor and refiner, and though we cannot see our ultimate potential when we look in the mirror, He sees us for who we will ultimately become.

If you feel you are far away from the presence of your Heavenly Father, you need only kneel down to feel closer. When you kneel in prayer, you figuratively step closer to the presence of God. Joseph Smith taught, "Having a knowledge of God, we begin to know how to approach Him, and how to ask so as to receive an answer. When we understand the character of God, and know how to come to Him, He begins to unfold the heavens to us, and to tell us all about it. When we are ready to come to Him, He is ready to come to us."[1]

It is very difficult for me to think of the trials of wanting children and not receiving them without feeling emotional. Remembering those times when all I wanted was to be a mother and my desire remained out of reach still brings tears to my eyes. How my heart pains when I think of the feelings I had of my own diminished worth. I thought that because I couldn't have children, I was unworthy in some regard. I felt so far from my Heavenly Father's presence, even though my Savior was carrying me through those darkest of days.

I understand now why I experienced the trials I did. I needed to learn that even if I was never able to have a successful pregnancy, I am still of infinite worth. I know now without a shadow of a doubt that my Heavenly Father loves me. My Savior gave His life for me. The trials I faced helped build my confidence in my Heavenly Father's plan and my sure knowledge of my individual worth. I know that although the path may seem unclear at times and the obstacles great, it is still the right path.

My visiting teacher shared something she had learned from a class. She said Jesus Christ loves me so much that even if I was the only person on the earth, He would have still fulfilled the Atonement. He would have died just for me, and that is exactly what He did. He died for each one of us because He knows our individual worth.

Regardless of how many children we have or do not have, we are of infinite worth. President James E. Faust said, "However, if children do not come, couples who are nevertheless prepared to receive them with love will be honored and blessed by the Lord for their faithfulness. Our homes should be among the most hallowed of all earthly sanctuaries."[2] Just as Abraham was promised, we are to become leaders on this earth in some way. We need to focus our lives so that we are ready to do what Heavenly Father needs when the time comes. Not all of our desires will be realized in this life.

Another scripture that offered me great peace, hope, and comfort during my trials was Doctrine and Covenants 121:7–9. When I read this scripture, I felt the Lord was speaking directly to me, saying, "My [daughter], peace be unto thy soul; thine adversity and thine afflictions shall be but a small moment; And then, if thou endure it well, God shall exalt thee on high; thou shalt triumph over all thy foes. Thy friends do stand by thee, and they shall hail thee again with warm hearts and friendly hands." Although this scripture was originally given to the Prophet Joseph in Liberty Jail, I felt I could give my own meaning to verse 9 to imply that my lost children were standing by me. I still feel that they are cheering me on in the heavens. And if I am not able to bring them all to this earth for the time I desired, I may see them again, and they will greet me with warm hearts and friendly hands and call out, "Mother."

How to Find Joy during Our Wait for Promised Blessings

One of my Gospel Doctrine teachers once shared the following with me.

> All trials make us bitter or better. This is my opinion, based upon what I learned after teaching Gospel Doctrine. Before we came here, we agreed to deal with whatever trials and tests the Lord would give us as an opportunity to be shaped into what we needed to become like Him. We were willing and we wanted it.
>
> If we could somehow convince the Lord to take away the trial, thereby taking away our growth from a trial, we might one day stand before Him and say, "You mean you took away the very trial that would perfect me?"

This is why our Heavenly Father will not take away our trials. We need them to qualify for eternal life. He allows us to have trials and then offers to strengthen us to be able to bear those burdens. Like Joseph Smith in Liberty Jail, we must also rise above our afflictions, no matter what our circumstances are.

Carmen shared how she felt when she dealt with a period of infertility.

> My good friend and neighbor had her twins on Sunday. She had two baby girls, and the babies are doing well. I am so happy for them, but a small part of me is a bit jealous. I know I shouldn't have those feelings, but they announced they were pregnant the same time we started trying, so if things would have gone normally, I would be having a baby soon. Sometimes I think Heavenly Father is not going to let me have another baby until I am more patient and loving to the ones I have. And sometimes I think Heavenly Father knows the best time for us.

Sheri Dew is an excellent example to me of someone who understands our Father in Heaven's plan. She has served in many great capacities and shows a defining sense of her womanly role although she remains unmarried. I sense in her a direction that many in her same situation lack. She knows she is of infinite worth, no matter what blessings are not yet obtained during this brief sojourn on earth.

Sometimes, amid all of our pain and trials, we become confused. It is hard to see the path that we must trod. My dad is a truck driver who has driven over a million miles in the last twenty-five years, and he has never been in an accident. With all the accidents that happen every year, how has my dad remained unscathed? Because he knows the road, and he knows where the road leads. He is not a long-haul driver. Instead, he drives the same route day after day and week after week, with little variation. He pays attention to landmarks and his surroundings and is aware of how the road moves through the regions he travels.

Several years ago, I rode home with my parents through a terrible blizzard. As we approached the mountain pass, we wondered if the road might be closed. The snow was drifting everywhere to the point that we could neither see the road nor the white line that separated us from the shoulder, which dropped off in many places into a shallow embankment.

It was frightening because we were driving very slowly and kept seeing vehicles off the road.

My dad kept a positive attitude and kept our worries at bay as he explained to us that we would be all right because he knew the road. He described to us how as we started uphill, the road would sweep wide to the right, and then a little later it would wind to the left. We stopped a few times to check on other cars that had slid off the road and were stuck in three feet of snow. We couldn't help much because we were only in a car, but we tried to check to see that they were okay. As we continued on, though I still could not see the road and everywhere I looked was blanketed in white, I knew we would be safe because my dad knew the way.

Heavenly Father has revealed the way to all of us. The path is strait and narrow and filled with difficult obstacles, yet we have been commanded to follow it. Sometimes it may be a struggle to know where we are headed, even as we grasp tightly to the iron rod. But if we will come to "know the way" of our Heavenly Father, we will be able to stay on the path that eventually leads to Him. He has given us the tools we need to learn the way. Through prayer, scripture study, and church and temple attendance, we can learn where our path leads us and also how to be prepared when it takes a sudden curve or something stands in our way.

My dad knew the way along that snow-covered road and led us safely home. Heavenly Father is willing to show us the way, and through our belief in Him and Jesus Christ, we can be led safely home as well.

It is my hope that this book has helped you to understand how much love your Father in Heaven has for you, despite the trials you face. I would like to share the song I wrote for my firstborn child, my daughter, not long after she was born. When I wrote these words, I was so grateful to finally be a mother, but I was also eternally grateful for the knowledge that God's hand is in our lives and that each of us are of infinite worth.

MY SONG FOR GRACIE

"Please, God, give me grace,"
I whispered in a prayer.
"Lift me up from this place
"Help me escape my despair."

"Please God, give me grace.
"Let me be a mother."
For years this phrase
was all that I could utter.

"Oh, please, God, give me grace.
"Look down from heaven and answer my prayers.
"Please give me grace
"I need hope 'cause life's not fair."

All I wanted was a baby.
Twice I almost thought they'd come,
But I was kept waiting
Praying for a daughter or a son.

And then God gave me Grace
Sent from heaven to answer my prayers.
God gave me Grace
With her blue eyes and blonde hair.

God gave me Grace.
How I love her so.
Each day I look at her
I know
God gave me Grace.

He heard my plea,
He helped me see.
God gave me Grace.

Notes:

1. Joseph Smith, *Teachings of the Prophet Joseph Smith*, comp. Joseph Fielding Smith (Salt Lake City: Deseret Book, 1976), 40–41.
2. James E. Faust, "Enriching Your Marriage," *Ensign*, April 2007, 8.

chapter 11

FREQUENTLY ASKED QUESTIONS

1.   Why did this happen to me?

Remember, we are all of infinite worth, and we will all experience specific trials during this lifetime. Miscarriages are a common occurrence, but your experience with miscarriage and how you deal with it will be unique to you. There is no one specific reason that will answer all "why" questions, but if you will have faith and rely on the Lord, in time you will come to learn from your trials. One reason I believe this happened to you was so that you could comfort others. If we never went through any trials, how could we empathize with each other? I encourage you to recognize your own possibilities for growth as you overcome your trials. Read Chapter 2 to learn more.

2.   How soon can I try to get pregnant again?

See the section "Getting Pregnant Again" in Chapter 4 on page 29.

3.   How can I overcome the fear of trying again?

See Chapter 4.

4.   How can I face everyone after announcing it?

See chapter 3, specifically the section "Don't Talk to Me! Everything Hurts!" on page 17.

5. How can I get the desire to go back to church?
See Chapter 4, especially "Staying Actively Engaged" on page 27.

6. How can I help my family understand what I'm going through?
See Chapters 1 and 3.

7. Do I have a celestial baby to raise in the hereafter?
See Chapter 2.

8. Is the Lord punishing me for something I did wrong?
See Chapters 1, 5, and 10.

9. How do I keep from feeling bitter about my circumstances?
See Chapter 10.

10. How can I get on with life?
See Chapter 3 and 4.

11. What should I do when people ask nosy questions?
See Chapter 3.

12. How can I help others who are going through similar situations?

One of my close friends has experienced four consecutive miscarriages. I'm thankful she was willing to share some of the things that have helped her. She said,

> Here are some helpful things that were given to me:
>
> • A plant so I could tend it and watch it grow—just a reminder of the baby. I don't have a grave to go to, but this is something I can remember the babies by.
> • A blanket for me and my husband to cuddle up in—a way for us to be together.
> • My mom and sister made me a baby box. My friend had to deliver her baby at five months because there was no heartbeat. The hospital gave her a box to remember the baby by. It contained a blanket and a stuffed animal, a journal, a baby bootie, and a camera to take a

picture of the baby. My mom and sister put a white baby blanket, a white hat, and a white stuffed animal in the box. This brought comfort to me. It was a way to not forget that there was a baby.

+ One friend gave me a white handkerchief so I could mourn the babies gone too soon.

+ I had a friend bring me a baby blanket so I could someday hold my baby.

13. Could I have done something to prevent this?
See Chapter 1.

14. How common are miscarriages?
See Chapter 1.

15. What kinds of tests are available to diagnose my problem?
Because early first-trimester miscarriages are very common and extensive testing is time-consuming and expensive, many doctors will not order any tests or see any cause for alarm with the first miscarriage. Usually it is only after a patient experiences three or more consecutive miscarriages, that the doctors begin testing to try to discover the problem.

There are a multitude of tests available, but because of the many unknowns involved with miscarriage, some tests may not be given unless you have experienced several miscarriages. For example, there is a test that can identify antiphospholipid syndrome (APS), but the test is costly and lengthy, and because the condition is rare, it is not the first choice for testing. I spoke with one woman who has had four miscarriages and was very recently diagnosed with APS because she requested her blood be tested. Another woman had a progesterone deficiency that caused two miscarriages before a doctor discovered the problem.

It would be most helpful for you to be in tune with your individual health, diet, and body. Make an effort to be healthy. Take vitamin supplements, exercise, and be as aware of your health as possible.

16. Do you know of any studies or other resources available?
The EAGeR study is an ongoing study that is being conducted by a group of universities and includes 1600 women who have suffered a miscarriage. The purpose of the study is to review the effects of low-dose

aspirin taken before pregnancy and continuing throughout pregnancy. To learn more about this study visit its website at www.eagertrial.org.

October is National Pregnancy and Infant Loss Awareness Month so there may be specific events in your area during that month.

There are several support groups via the Internet that you can join to talk to others suffering from similar problems. One such organization is "Share Pregnancy & Infant Loss Support, Inc," which you can access at http://www.nationalshare.org/index.html.

Other books you can read to help:

- *If God Loves Me, Why This? Finding Peace in God's Plan for Us* by Kim A. Nelson
- *Unsung Lullaby* by Josi Kilpack
- *To Love and to Promise* by Rachel Ann Nunes
- *The Birth We Call Death* by Paul H. Dunn and Richard M. Eyre
- *Never, Never Will She Stop Loving You* by Jolene Durrant
- *We Were Gonna Have a Baby, but We Had an Angel Instead* by Pat Schwiebert, illustrated by Taylor Bills

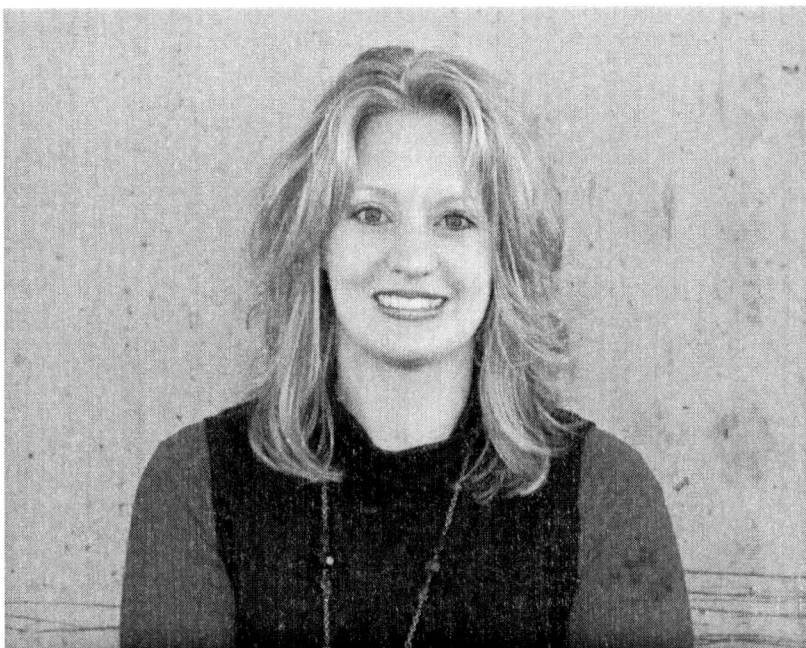

aBOUT THE aUTHOR

Rachelle J. Christensen was born and raised in a small farming town in Idaho. Her creativity developed easily in this rural area since she spent many years working in the fields with only a few weeds to distract her daydreaming. She graduated cum laude from Utah State University with a bachelor's degree in psychology and a minor in music. Rachelle loves spending time with her family and writing during every spare minute she has. She also enjoys singing and songwriting, playing the piano, running, motivational speaking, and—of course—reading.

Rachelle has created a special musical fireside based on *Lost Children*; you can visit her website, www.rachellechristensen.com, for information on how to schedule a presentation. You can also visit Rachelle at her blog: www.rachellewrites.blogspot.com.